Y

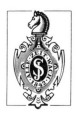

H. Bismuth   D. Castaing

# Operative Ultrasound of the Liver and Biliary Ducts

With 69 Figures

Springer-Verlag
Berlin Heidelberg New York
London Paris Tokyo

Professor Dr. Henri Bismuth
Professor Dr. Denis Castaing
Unité de Chirurgie Hépato-biliaire
et Département de Chirurgie Expérimentale
Hôpital Paul Brousse
et Université Paris-Sud
UER médicale Kremlin Bicêtre
F-94800 Villejuif

Translation of:
Bismuth/Castaing, Echographie per-operative du foie et des voies biliaires
© 1985 by Flammarion Paris, France
ISBN 2-257-10440-4

ISBN 3-540-17091-X Springer-Verlag Berlin Heidelberg New York
ISBN 0-387-17091-X Springer-Verlag New York Berlin Heidelberg

Library of Congress Cataloging-in-Publication Data. Bismuth, H. Operative ultrasound of the liver and biliary
ducts. Translation of: Echographie per-operatoive du foie et des voies biliaires. Includes bibliographies.
1. Liver − Surgery. 2. Biliary ducts − Surgery. 3. Diagnosis, Ultrasonic. I. Castaing, D. II. Title. [DNLM:
1. Biliary Tract − surgery. 2. Liver − surgery. 3. Ultrasonic Diagnosis. WI 770 B62225e]
RD546.B5513   1987   617′.556   86-31614
ISBN 0-387-17091-X (U.S.)

Typesetting and printing: Petersche Druckerei GmbH & Co. Offset KG, 8803 Rothenburg ob der Tauber
Bookbinding: Konrad Triltsch, Graphischer Betrieb, 8700 Würzburg
2121/3130-543210

# Contents

# Introduction

Operative ultrasound, which permits direct placement of the probe on the organ to be studied during surgery, has been in existence for over 20 years. Early experiences with its use in urologic [15] and biliary surgery [7, 8, 9] were limited by technical difficulties but the evolution of B-mode, real-time ultrasound has made possible the broad application of ultrasound in the operating room.

The goal of operative ultrasound is to provide the surgeon with information about a solid organ which is not obvious from its external morphology. What is the nature of the lesion? What is its precise localization within the organ? What vascular and anatomical constraints limit its surgical treatment? Modern ultrasound technology, which produces an image faithful to the true anatomy, permits the surgeon to answer these questions intraoperatively.

Multiple successful experiences with operative ultrasound have been reported, first in urologic surgery [1, 6], then in biliary surgery with the work of Lane [10, 11] and Sigel [16], and in hepatic surgery by Makuuchi and Hasegawa [13]. In pancreatic surgery, advances have been reported in the detection of small lesions by Lane [4] and Chapuis [12]. Reports of many other successful applications have been published in other fields of surgery [2, 5, 14, 17].

This book is the result of more than 2 years of intensive application of operative ultrasound [3] by a team of hepatobiliary surgeons (H. Bismuth, D. Castaing, and D. Houssin). During our early experience we benefitted from the help of a radiologist, F. Kunstlinger. Our goal has been the development of a practical guide for those who wish to apply operative ultrasound in the surgical treatment of hepatobiliary diseases.

We have divided the material into three principal sections: hepatic surgery, biliary surgery, and the surgery of portal hypertension. Our experience with operative ultrasound in pancreatic disease is not adequate for discussion in this manual, although many useful applications have been suggested. Each chapter includes an anatomical review and a presentation of the basic sonographic signs to clarify the diagnosis and therapy of pathologic conditions. Emphasis has been placed on the practical applications of operative ultrasound.

With most of the ultrasound images (all are presented on a black background) two schematic diagrams are shown:

The first indicates the position of the probe on anterior and lateral projections.
The second is a diagram of the image which highlights the essential details. Hyperechoic regions are white, while hypoechoic areas are in black.

## References

1. Andaloro VA, Schor M, Marangola JP (1976) Intraoperative localization of renal calculi using ultrasound. J Urol 116:92–93
2. Belghiti J, Menu Y, Nahum H, et al (1984) Apport de l'echographie per-opératoire dans la chirurgie des tumeurs du foie. Presse Med 13: 1839–1841
3. Bismuth H, Castaing D, Kunstlinger F (1984) L'échographie per-opératoire en chirurgie hépato-biliaire. Presse Med 13:1819–1822
4. Chapuis Y, Hernigou A, Poirier A, et al (1983) Détection échographique en temps réel per-opératoire d'un insulinome pancréatique. Presse Med 12:2535–2536
5. Chapuis Y, Hernigou A, Plainfosse MC, et al (1984) Exemples d'application de l'ultrasonographie temps réel per-opératoire en chirurgie endocrinienne. Chirurgie 110:97–104

2

6. Cook UH, Lytton B (1977) Intraoperative localization of renal calculi during nephrolithothomy by ultrasound scanning. J Urol 117:543–546
7. Eiseman B, Greenlaw RH, Gallagher JG (1965) Localization of common duct stones by ultrasound. Arch Surg 91:195–199
8. Hayaski S, Wagai T, Miyazawa R (1962) Ultrasonic diagnosis of breast tumour and cholelithiasis. West J Surg Obstet Gynecol 70:34–36
9. Knight PR, Newell JA (1963) Operative use of ultrasonics in cholelithiasis. Lancet i:1023–1025
10. Lane RJ, Crocker EF (1979) Operative ultrasonic bile duct scanning. Anat NZJ Surg 49:454–458
11. Lane RJ, Glazer G (1980) Intraoperative B-mode ultrasound scanning of the extrahepatic biliary tree and pancreas. Lancet i:334–337
12. Lane RJ, Coupland GAE (1982) Operative ultrasonic features of insulinomas. Am J Surg 144:595–597
13. Makuuchi M, Hasegawa H, Yamazaki S (1981) Intraoperative ultrasonic examination for hepatectomy. Jap J Clin Oncol 11:367–389
14. Plainfosse MC, Merran S (1983) Intraoperative abdominal ultrasound. Radiology 147:829–833
15. Schlebel JO, Diggdon P, Cuellar J (1961) The use of ultrasound for localizing renal calculi. J Urol 86:367–369
16. Sigel B, Spigos DG, Donahue PE, et al (1979) Intraoperative ultrasonic visualisation of biliary calculi. Curr Surg 36:158–159
17. Sigel B (1982) Operative ultrasonography. Lea and Fibiger, Philadelphia

# 1 General Considerations in Operative Ultrasound

## How Is the Ultrasound Image Formed?

Sounds are pressure waves which are propagated at variable speeds, depending on the elastic properties of the medium in which they are travelling. These pressure waves produce a reflection on striking an obstacle (an interface between two mediums with different elastic properties), which can be sensed by a receiving device. These reflections are termed echoes.

Ultrasound waves are high-frequency signals which exceed 15000 cycles per second (15000 Hz). Ultrasound frequencies used in abdominal scanning vary from $2 \times 10^6$ to $10 \times 10^6$ Hz or 2 to 10 MHz. This range of frequencies is not chosen arbitrarily, but is limited by the following physical constraints:

1. The primary goal in scanning is to obtain the greatest possible precision; i.e., to identify the smallest possible objects. For physical reasons the smallest detail one can observe is of the order of several multiples of the wavelength being utilized. (In water the maximal resolution is 0.5 mm per 3 MHz.) The use of a short wavelength implies a high frequency, since they have an inverse relationship.
2. The maximal wavelength which can be used is limited by the loss of energy by the signal as it passes through the medium, a loss which increases with increasing frequency. For these reasons, the depth of the area which can be scanned is limited by the frequency of the signal.

For scanning, the ideal system must represent a compromise between two opposing factors. Since operative ultrasound permits the placement of the probe directly on the organ to be scanned, it allows greater accuracy than percutaneous scanning. A higher-frequency signal is used, since the sound wave does not have to travel through the layers of the abdominal wall.

The probe, termed a transducer, is both a transmitter and a receiver of the ultrasound signal. It is applied directly to the surface of the organ to be scanned and emits an ultrasound beam of short duration. After the emission the transducer receives the echoes, which are then transformed into electrical signals and presented as points on a cathode ray screen by the pulse-processing system. The position of the point on the screen is proportional to the amount of time which elapses between emission and reception, and therefore represents the distance between the probe and the structure being visualized. The brightness of the point on the screen, which ranges from white to black through a spectrum of grey, is related to the amplitude of the reflection. This is called B-mode ultrasound.

There are two different imaging techniques:

1. In contact ultrasound, the image is constructed one line at a time. Time is required to form and fix each image.
2. In real-time ultrasound, the probe is constructed with multiple transducers, whose firing sequence is coordinated in a continuous cycle. This permits the immediate reconstruction of the image and thus the possibility of dynamic imaging.

Two types of probe exist for real-time imaging:

1. If the multiple transducers have a linear arrangement, an image is produced which is composed of multiple parallel lines and forms a wide sweep.

4

2. If the transducers have a radial arrangement, a sector scan is produced which constructs a pie-shaped image. A similar image can be produced by a single transducer either with a set of mirrors or a motor which rapidly moves the transducer through an arc.

In both cases a cross-sectional image is produced of the area being scanned. The image reconstructed on the cathode ray screen can be reproduced on photographic film or on video tape. By convention the images are recorded using white on a black background with the upper portion of the image representing the area closest to the probe. In transverse sections the left of the image corresponds to the patient's right (Fig. 1). In longitudinal sections, the left is superior, the right inferior.

## Operation of the Ultrasound Equipment

### The Gain Curve

Depending on the frequency of the ultrasound beam and the characteristics of the medium, a progressive loss of energy occurs with increasing depth. This loss of energy is a function of the density of the medium. Modern ultrasound equipment compensates for this attenuation by using a system which regulates the intensity of the beam as a function of the depth of imaging. This regulation, which is termed time-gain compensation, varies in complexity between different types of equipment: near gain, far gain, overall gain, and the slope of the gain curve (dB/cm). These are simple systems which are controlled manually. More complex systems can provide a continuous modification of gain during imaging. This regulation is of fundamental importance for obtaining interpretable images: for good imaging a gain setting is chosen which produces a uniform tone of grey over the entire depth of an area of homogeneous echodensity (Fig. 2).

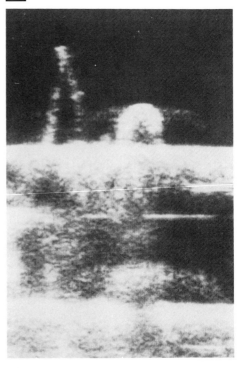

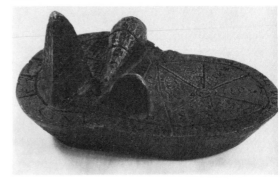

**Fig. 1. A** The ultrasound image is not a strict reconstruction of the object as it appears in reality, but rather a representation of the acoustic interfaces which reflect or refract sound waves depending on their intrinsic properties. **B** The liver of Piacenza, an Etruscan model, more than 2000 years old

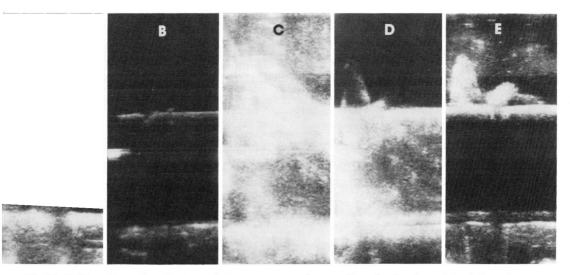

**Fig. 2A–E.** The settings of a pulse-processing system must produce a uniform density of grey through the entire depth of the scan (**A**). In **B** the gain is too weak, resulting in a loss of detail. In **C** the total gain is set too high, creating images which obscure the shape of the object being scanned. In **D** the far gain is set too high, while in **E** the near gain is excessive, producing a distorted image in both cases

6

When the beam crosses an sonolucent (liquid) region which is surrounded by normal parenchyma, the automatic compensation for depth will produce an intensification of the the signal in the region beyond the liquid zone, since little energy is lost by the signal as it traverses liquid. By contrast, when the beam encounters an interface between areas of differing impedence, scatter will occur which will cause a reduction in intensity, or attenuation, of the beam. Highly attenuating structures such as calculi will completely arrest the progress of the ultrasound beam and produce an acoustic shadow distally (Fig. 3). Since air transmits almost no signal, it produces an effect similar to calculi and can be a source of diagnostic confusion. Slight variation of the total gain can sometimes clarify these modifications.

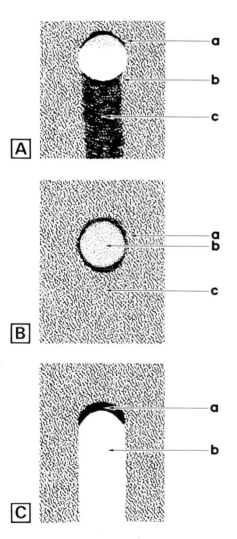

◀ **Fig. 3A–C.** Ultrasound images. **A** Sonolucent structure of liquid density: in *a* the upper border is visible. Note the small artefacts which appear as the gain is increased. The lateral borders are not visible. Beginning at the back wall *(b)*, posterior accentuation is seen *(c)*, since little energy is lost as the beam traverses a liquid medium. **B** Solid structure producing a hypoechoic image. All the edges have a uniform density *(a)*, the echoes are equally distributed within the mass *(b)*, and there is no posterior accentuation *(c)*. **C** Shadowing structure containing calcium. Only the anterior surface is visible. The image is intense *(a)* and the beam does not proceed beyond the object *(b)*. This effect is termed an acoustic shadow

## Other Modes of Regulation

*1. Focusing.* Resolution along the axis of the ultrasound beam is related to the wavelength, whereas resolution perpendicular to the axis is related to the width of the beam, which can be varied using a sort of acoustic lens to improve imaging at different depths.

*2. The other types of regulation* are of little practical interest for operative ultrasound.

## Choice of Equipment

The equipment should ideally be simple to use while providing a high-quality image. The discussion of equipment is organized under the following headings: the pulse-processing system, the transducer probe, and ancillary equipment for biopsy or other manipulations.

### Pulse-Processing Systems

B-mode, real-time scanning is essential, as it demonstrates respiratory and hemodynamic variations and is sensitive to slight movements of the probe. Static scanning is not practical for operating room use.

Linear scanning is preferable to sectoral scanning, as the image is not deformed and location of the structures can be directly related to the position of the probe.

We have used two systems: Aloka model SSD 256 (distributed in France by AHS, 95004 Cergy-Pontoise Cedex) and Scanel 500 CGR (Ultra-Sonic, 77102 Meaux). Both systems use linear scanning, and neither is specifically designed for operating room use.

The equipment should be portable and not occupy too much space in the operating room. Gain and focusing are the only functions that are essential for routine operative ultrasound.

### The Transducer Probe

Proper choice of this device is essential for successful operative ultrasound. The probe must be waterproof and completely sterilizable, including the connecting wire for the pulse processor, The size and shape of the probe are important. For the Aloka system we have used the UST 582 I 5 and UST 582 T 5 heads of 5 MHz and measuring $7 \times 2 \times 1.5$ cm. For the CGR system, SLOT 5 and SLOT 7.5 are used, which are of 5 and 7.5 MHz and measure $7 \times 2 \times 0.7$ cm.

For the liver a T-shaped probe is useful, as it can easily be placed at the hilus and fits between the liver and the diaphragm (Fig. 4). A frequency of 5 MHz permits a scanning depth of 5–10 cm, which is adequate for intra-abdominal scanning.

For the extrahepatic bile ducts a straight probe is easier to use. Frequencies of 7.5 or even 10 MHz are used, since a shallow scanning depth is adequate.

### Ancillary Equipment

Immediately beneath the probe is a zone which is not well visualized. This zone varies in depth between probes, but is usually 5 mm. This limitation is overcome by the use of a water pouch, which is placed between the probe and the structure to be scanned. A distance of 1–2 cm will provide good visualization. The water pouch should be thin-walled and contain a homogeneous liquid free of air bubbles. A condom filled with water is ideal for this purpose.

A guide for the biopsy needle is necessary to accurately puncture small structures (less than 1 cm). We use a Plexiglas guide which fits directly onto the probe. The angle of puncture can be varied between 30°, 45°, and 60°. The guide is designed so that the needle can be removed from it at any time to facilitate manipulation. In addition, using the cursors for making measurements on the screen, further control over the puncture axes is provided by direct visualization of the needle on the screen as the biopsy is performed.

We use various needles depending upon their application:

For biopsies, automatic Menghini needles with a gauge of 18–20 (Hépafix type)

For punctures and subsequent injection, 22-gauge Chiba needles

For punctures with catheterization, Teflon-coated needles initially designed for translumbar aortography (18-gauge)

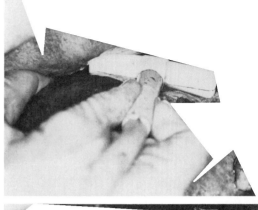

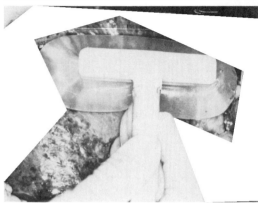

**Fig. 4A, B.** The Aloka UST 582 T-S probe, of 5 Mhz, is applied **A** directly to the surface of the liver or **B** with the water pouch

## Technique of Operative Ultrasound

### Sterilization of Equipment

Sterilization of the equipment has not been a significant problem. The chassis can be sterilized with the same level of care as the operating room or other radiographic equipment.

We have used several methods for the sterilization of the probe and cable. Sterilization with ethylene oxide is probably the best method; however, the long duration of the process necessitates the possession of a large number of probes. Cold sterilization in formalin (12 h) or in Chlorhexidine (Hibitane) or povidone-iodine (for at least 20 min) is acceptable and more practical. In all cases the probe should be rinsed in sterile saline before intraoperative use. Monthly cultures of equipment sterilized with these techniques have shown no evidence of contamination.

An alternative method of handling this problem is to wrap the probe in a long sterile plastic bag which is filled with transmitting gel. This system is slightly less convenient, but it avoids the technical problems of sterilization of the probe.

### Utilization of Equipment

The sterile probe is placed in the operative field with the cord being passed off to the circulating nurse and connected to the pulse-processing system. To obtain maximum length, the system should be placed near the operating table. A television screen can be used to project the image for more convenient viewing.

Since the surgeon is not able to regulate the image himself, the system must be simple to operate. The surgeon manipulates the probe directly, keeping it, directly or with a water pouch, in contact with the organ being studied (Fig. 4). The operative field can be filled with saline to act as a medium for certain types of scanning.

The probe should be moved slowly and systematically with small rotational movements for optimal reconstruction of the three-dimensional structure of the regions being scanned. A record of the images obtained is made on film, polaroid film, or videotape.

# 2 Operative Ultrasound in Hepatic Surgery

## Technique of Exploration

### Incisions

The liver can be examined through any incision which permits the surgeon's hand to be placed between the liver and the diaphragm. Adhesions or displacement of the round ligament to the right by hepatic atrophy are factors which can interfere with a proper examination. In general, however, the liver can be studied thoroughly even through an infraumbilical midline incision.

### Methodology

The exploration of the liver is performed by placing the probe directly on the surface of the liver, whose natural humidity permits ultrasound examination without the use of a transmitting gel. Gentle pressure is necessary to maintain good contact, but excessive pressure should be avoided as it will distort the image by collapsing vascular structures. The probe is moved slowly, using a slight rotational motion which permits reconstruction of the three-dimensional structure of the elements being studied [6, 17]. The superficial parenchyma of the liver represents a blind zone for the probe, and must be studied either with a water pouch or by placing the probe on the other side of the liver. (A condom filled with water is ideal for this purpose as it is thin-walled and flexible. When using the pouch the gain setting must be altered to obtain a good image.)

### Exploration (Fig. 5)

The same sequence should be followed each time to ensure a thorough examination

(Fig. 5). The hepatic veins are examined first at their junction with the vena cava. The probe should be placed on the anterior surface of the liver with a slight superior inclination. Turning the probe to the right or the left will direct the ultrasound beam parallel with the course of the hepatic veins, which can then be examined along their entire course as far as their tributaries, even when the latter are only 2–3 mm in diameter.

The exploration is then continued by examining the portal pedicles. The probe is still on the anterior surface of the liver, but is moved slightly lower, near the anterior edge. The examination begins on the left near the round ligament, then proceeds toward the right past the hilus and into the right side of the liver, where the branches of the portal pedicles can be identified and followed. Within these pedicles the biliary radicles, the portal vein branches, and the hepatic arterial branches are visible. The location of these structures, which are of critical importance in hepatic surgery, can then be marked on the surface of the liver with electrocautery. The parenchyma is examined last, and should be studied in its entirety, with the aid of water pouch.

The systematic study of the liver is followed by examination of the gallbladder and the hepatoduodenal ligament. These are studied either directly with the water pouch or through the hepatic parenchyma.

## Ultrasound Anatomy of the Liver

We use the nomenclature of Couinaud [5] (Fig. 6). Thirty patients with normal livers were studied during abdominal operations

12

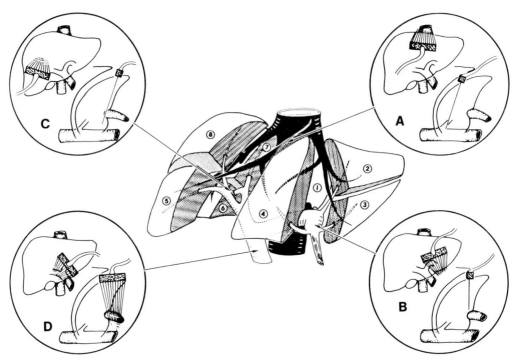

**Fig. 5A–D.** Technique of ultrasound examination of the liver. **A** Examination of the hepatic veins: the probe is placed horizontally on the anterior surface of the liver and oriented with a slight superior inclination. **B** The probe is placed anteriorly and inferiorly and tilted toward the *left* for examination of the left portal pedicle and its branches. **C** The probe is moved toward the *right* to visualize the right portal pedicle and its branches. **D** The transhepatic study of the hilus can be performed with the probe held either horizontally or vertically. For definition of segments *1–8*, see Fig. 6

not related to the liver or the biliary tree. They provide the basis for the anatomical study.

**The Inferior Vena Cava and the Hepatic Veins**

The vena cava is a longitudinal structure to the right of the midline. It appears as an echo-free band with sharp borders, and its diameter is seen to vary with respiration. The vena cava is posterior to the liver and does not indent its parenchyma.

The junction of the hepatic veins with the vena cava is usually easy to identify. The hepatic veins are external to Glisson's capsule and appear in the hepatic parenchyma as sonolucent spaces. The walls of these veins are difficult to see, as they appear as thin echogenic lines. Blood flow can be seen within the lumen of the veins as fine echoes. The cardiac pulsations are also transmitted to the hepatic veins, and this feature facilitates their identification [4].

In 26 out of 30 cases (86%), the left and middle hepatic veins join the vena cava as a common trunk (Fig. 7). Less commonly, three separate insertions are identified (Fig. 8).

The left hepatic vein is formed from multiple venous tributaries; in most cases (20 out of 30 – 67%) a large posterior trunk with multiple small anterior branches is seen. The main trunk measures 2–3 cm in length.

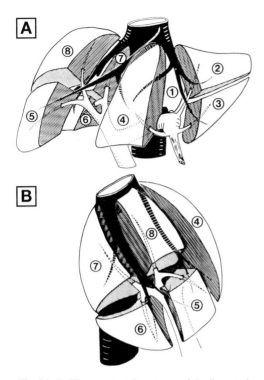

**Fig. 6A, B.** The segmental anatomy of the liver as described by Couinaud [5]. **A** anterior view; **B** right lateral projection. Eight segments are defined: segment *1*, or the caudate lobe; segments *2* and *3*, which constitute the left lobe; and segment *4*, whose anterior portion is the quadrate lobe. Segments *2, 3*, and *4* comprise the left liver and are perfused by the left branch of the hepatic artery and the left portal vein. Segments *5* and *8* comprise the anterior portion of the right liver and are supplied by the right anterior portal pedicle. The right posterior portal pedicle supplies segments *6* and *7*. The right liver is thus comprised of an anterior and a posterior portion

The middle hepatic vein is formed from two anterior veins (from segments 4 and 5) at about the level of the hilus (24 out of 30 cases − 80%; Fig. 9). Its trunk is long (3–5 cm) and lies obliquely in a superior and slightly anterior direction. In 53% of cases (16 out of 30), a branch from the superior portion of segment 4 empties into the middle heptic vein, which can also receive a branch from segment 8 (2 out of 30 cases − 7%). The segment 8 branch can also empty directly into the vena cava (Fig. 10). The plane between the middle hepatic vein and the inferior vena cava divides the liver into two portions which have independent portal vascularization. This is the principal portal fissure, which defines the surgical right and left lobes (Fig. 11).

The insertion of the right hepatic vein is into the right border of the inferior vena cava, slightly inferior to the insertion of the other two hepatic veins. In 70% of cases (21 out of 30), there is a single large trunk superior and posterior to the liver along the insertion of the coronary ligament (Fig. 12). In 13% of cases (4 out of 30), an accessory hepatic vein joins the inferior vena cava (Fig. 13) at the level of the hilus [16]. The probe must be directed posteriorly and into the parenchyma to define the right portal fissure, which separates the anterior and posterior portions of the right lobe. This is virtually a coronal plane, which is oblique inferiorly and passes between the inferior vena cava and the right posterior portal pedicle (Fig. 14).

The hepatic veins of segment 1 are difficult to visualize in a normal liver because of their small size. There are usually three or four of them, and they insert into the left side of the vena cava (Fig. 15).

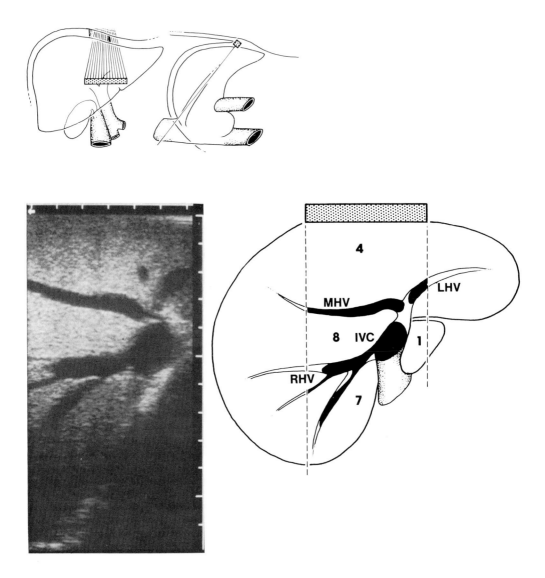

**Fig. 7.** Common insertion of the left *(LHV)*, and middle *(MHV)* hepatic vein into the inferior vena cava *(IVC)*. *RHV*, right hepatic vein. Transverse parenchymal section with a slight superior inclination

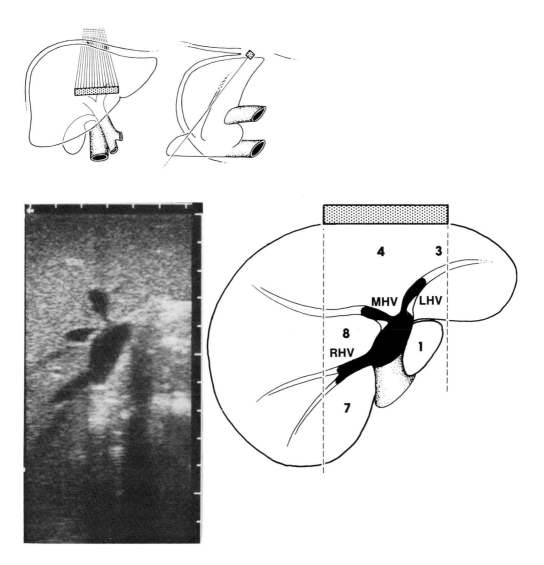

**Fig. 8.** Separate insertion of the three hepatic veins into the vena cava: left hepatic vein *(LHV)*, middle hepatic vein *(MHV)*, and right hepatic vein *(RHV)*. Transverse section with slight upward inclination to the right

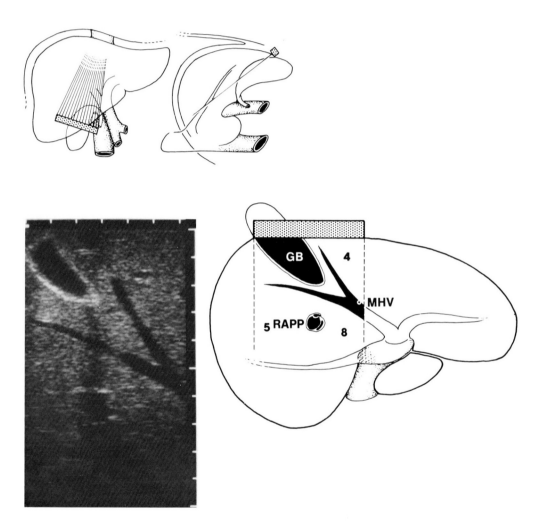

**Fig. 9.** Origin of the middle hepatic vein *(MHV)*, formed by the two anterior veins draining segments *4* and *5*. *GB*, gallbladder; *RAPP*, right anterior portal pedicle. Transverse section with a slight superior inclination near the anterior edge of the liver

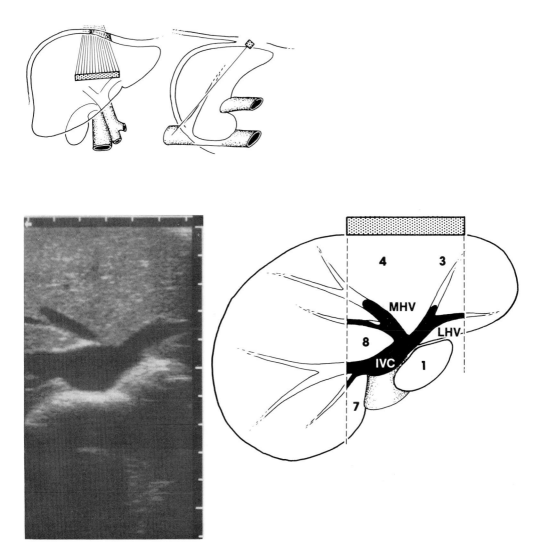

**Fig. 10.** The middle hepatic vein *(MHV)* receiving a branch from segment *8. LHV*, left hepatic vein. The three separate insertions of the hepatic veins into the vena cava *(IVC)* are also visible. Transverse section with a slight superior inclination

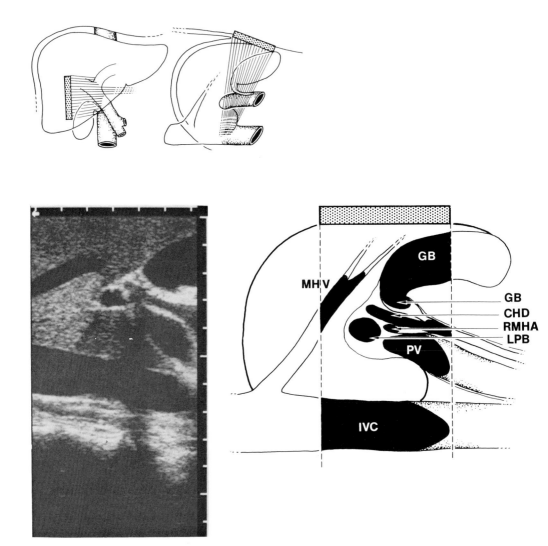

**Fig. 11.** Transhepatic sagittal section through the main portal fissure passing through the gallbladder *(GB)*, the hepatic pedicle with the main portal vein *(PV)*, the left portal branch *(LPB)*, and the common hepatic duct *(CHD)*, with the right middle hepatic artery *(RMHA)* passing between the main portal vein and the common hepatic duct. *IVC*, inferior vena cava; *MHK*, middle hepatic vein

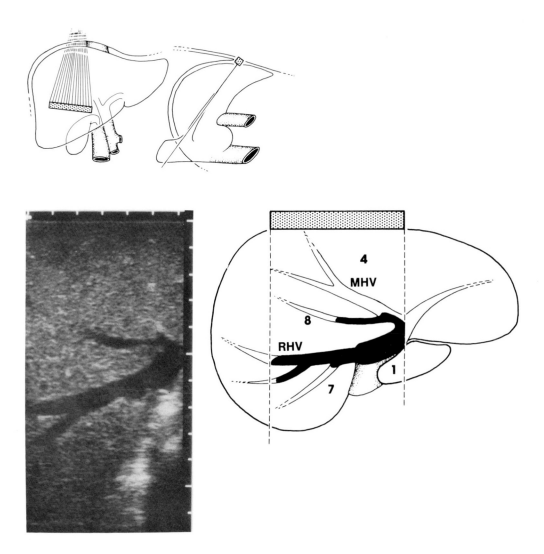

**Fig. 12.** Right hepatic vein *(RHV)* fed by several posterior branches. It joins the vena cava between segments *7* and *8*. The hepatic vein of segment *8* is visible as it empties into the middle hepatic vein *(MHV)*. Transverse section through the liver with a slight superior inclination

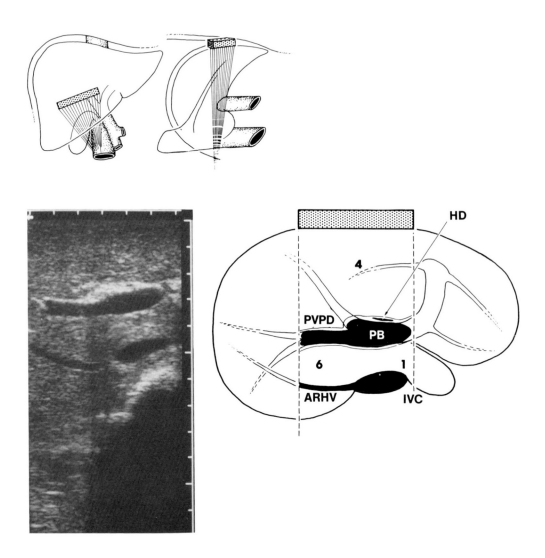

**Fig. 13.** Accessory right hepatic vein *(ARHV)* emptying into the inferior vena cava *(IVC)* inferiorly at the level of the hilus, at the junction of the right and left hepatic ducts *(HD)*, the portal bifurcation *(PB)*, and the right portal vein with its posterior division *(PVPD)*. Transverse transhepatic section at the level of the hilus

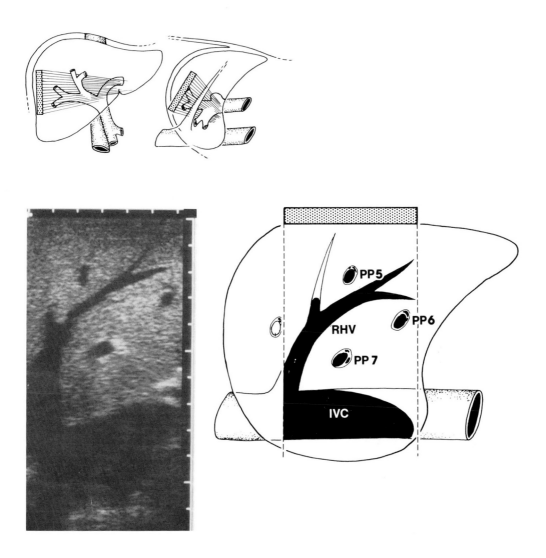

**Fig. 14.** Right portal fissure passing through the right hepatic vein *(RHV)*, the portal pedicle *(PP)*, of segment 5 (the inferior division of the right anterior pedicle) and those of segments 6 and 7 (right posterior pedicle), and the vena cava *(IVC)*. Coronal section passing through the vena cava

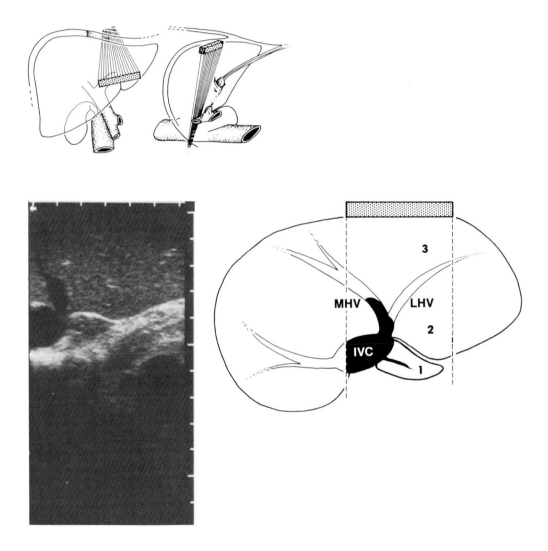

**Fig. 15.** The hepatic veins of segment *1* drain into the vena cava *(IVC)*. *MHV*, middle hepatic vein; *LHV*, left hepatic vein. Transverse transhepatic section inferior to the hilus

## The Portal Pedicles

The unit composed of the portal vein branch, the arterial branch, and the biliary radicle is enveloped in a fibrous sheath which is derived from Glisson's capsule. This capsule thickens at the hilus to become the hilar plate. With ultrasound this sheath is seen as a echogenic line which is much more dense than that surrounding the hepatic veins. The portal vein branch is the largest element within the portal pedicle. The branches of the hepatic artery are identified by their pulsations, which can be detected even in the most distal branches. The biliary radicle is often visualized deep in hepatic parenchyma, much deeper than in preoperative studies.

*The Hilus.* The portal bifurcation, which is extrahepatic, is easily recognized on a transverse section centered on the hilus and traversing the hepatic parenchyma (Fig. 16). The bile ducts are anterior and superior to the portal vein branches (Fig. 17). The arte-

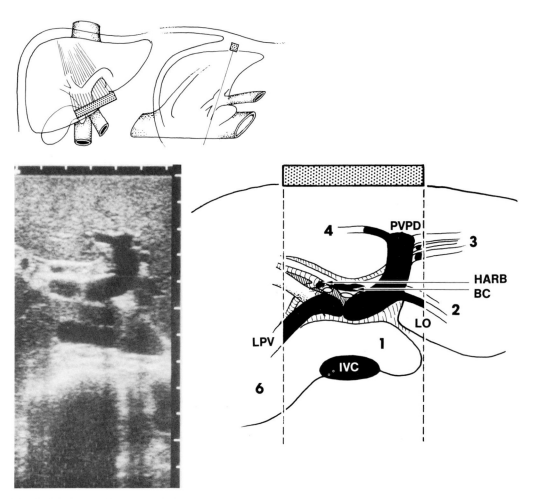

**Fig. 16.** The hilus with the portal bifurcation, the left portal vein *(LPV)* and the posterior division of the right portal vein *(PVPD)*, the arterial bifurcation with its right branch *(HARB)*, and the biliary convergence *(BC)*. *LO*, lesser omentum; *IVC*, vena cava. Transverse transhepatic section at the hilus

rial branches pass between the two and are sometimes difficult to see, as their bifurcation is lower and their course slightly different.

*The Left Portal Pedicle.* In the same plane, by moving the probe to the left, the left portal pedicle can be seen in its extrahepatic portion. Here it is possible to see the caudate branches (to segment 1), which exit posterior-

ly. In the same section, to the left, the portal vein branch crosses anteriorly to terminate as the recessus of Rex at the round ligament. It appears as a well-defined hyperechoic zone.

As the main portal vein turns posteriorly, it gives off the branch for segment 2. At the level of the recessus of Rex the portal branch divides into two one to the right for segment 4 and the other to the left for segment 3 (Fig. 18).

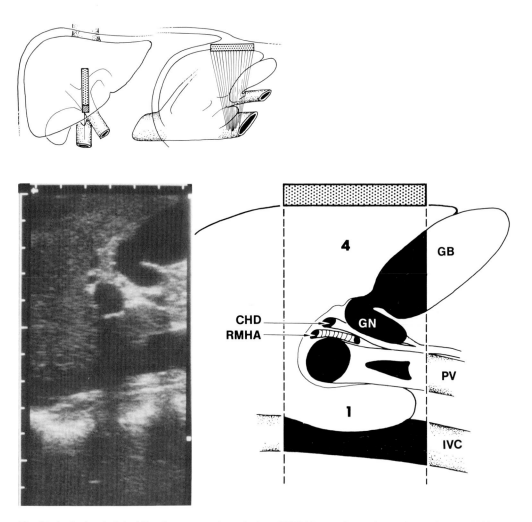

**Fig. 17.** At the level of the hilus the common hepatic duct *(CHD)* is anterior and superior to the portal bifurcation and the right branch of middle hepatic artery *(RMHA)*. It is contained within Glisson's capsule, which thickens to become the hilar plate, a structure which has a much greater echogenicity than the other hilar structures. *GN,* gallbladder neck; *PV,* portal vein; *IVC,* inferior vena cava. Longitudinal transhepatic section through the gallbladder *(GB)*

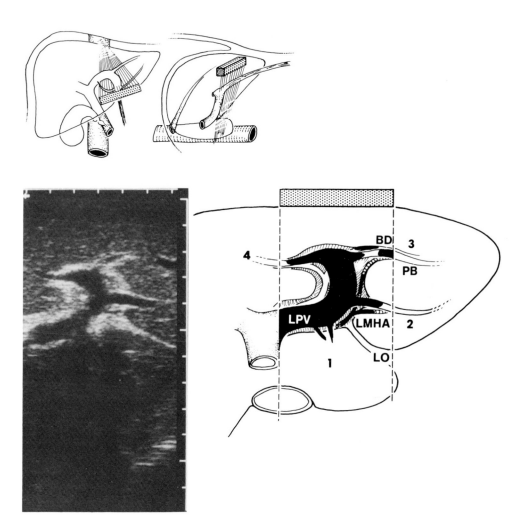

**Fig. 18.** Left portal pedicle containing the left portal vein *(LPV)*, the corresponding bile ducts *(BD)*, and the left branch of middle hepatic artery *(LMHA)* surrounded by the capsule. The extrahepatic portion is visible with its horizontal course in the highest part of the hilus. The intrahepatic portion is also visible with its anterior orientation, giving off the three pedicles to segments *2, 3*, and *4*. Note: the two portal branches *(PB)* to segment *1* originate from the extrahepatic portion of the left portal vein. *LO,* lesser omentum. Transverse section at the midline superior to the insertion of the round ligament

*The Right Portal Pedicle.* Leaving the hilus toward the right, the right portal vein branch is short and is directed superiorly. At a distance of 2 cm from the hilus it divides into two trunks (Fig. 19), one of which projects anteriorly to supply segments 5 and 8 between the middle and right hepatic veins (Figs. 20 and 21). The bile duct is localized by following the right portal vein branch and is usually (24 out of 30 cases − 80%) in an epiportal position, while the artery is in an inferior one.

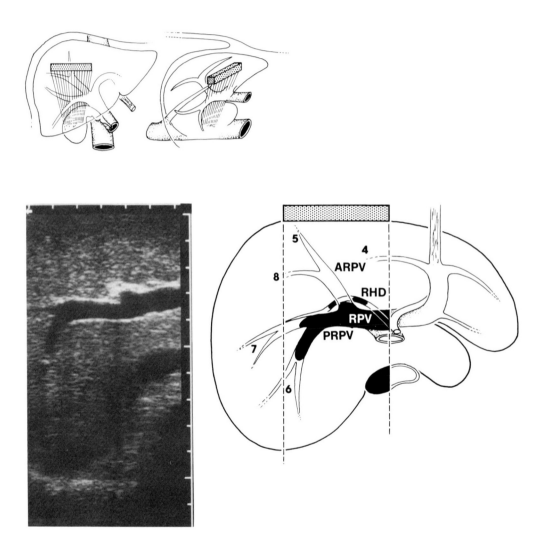

**Fig. 19.** The right portal vein *(RPV)* divides rapidly into two branches, an anterior one *(ARPV)* to segments 5 and 8, and a posterior division *(PRPV)* to segments 6 and 7. The right hepatic duct *(RHD)* is superior to the anterior branch of the right portal vein. Transverse section with a slightly superior inclination

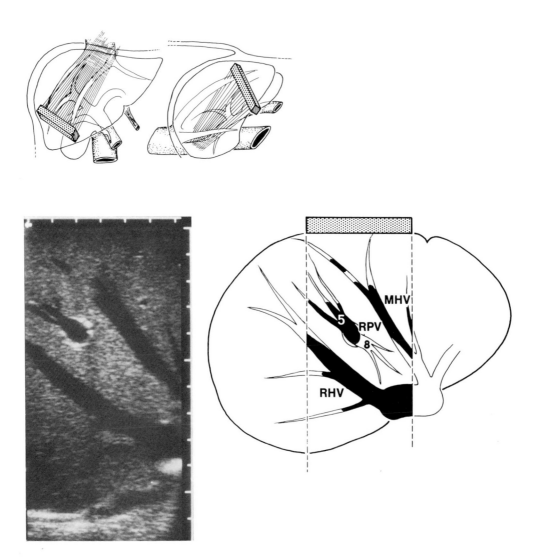

**Fig. 20.** The right anterior portal vein *(RPV)* divides into two segmental branches; the superior one to segment *8* and the inferior one to segment *5*. These vessels perfuse the anterior area of the right liver, which is bounded by the right *(RHV)* and middle *(MHV)* hepatic veins. Oblique section with a sharply superior inclination

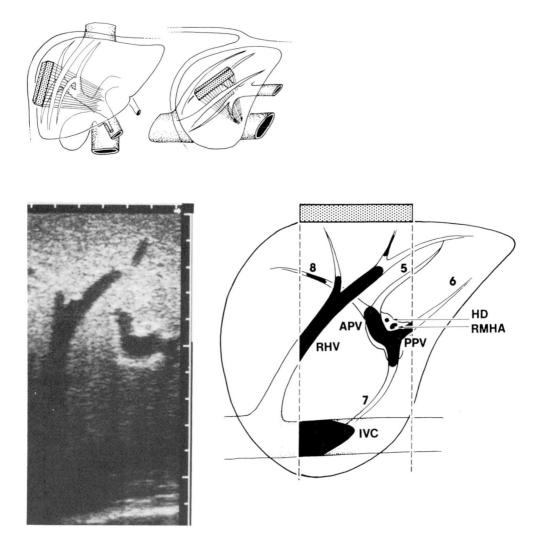

**Fig. 21.** The right portal vein has two sectoral branches: one proceeding anteriorly *(APV)* to segments 5 and 8, and the other posteriorly *(PPV)* to segments 6 and 7. The right hepatic vein *RHV)* courses between these four portal pedicles and with the vena cava *(IVC)* defines the right portal fissure. *HD*, hepatic duct; *RMHA*, right branch of the middle hepatic artery. Coronal posterior transhepatic section

The posterior trunk divides into branches for segments 6 and 7. Complete examination is not possible if the coronary ligament is large (Fig. 22). The position of the probe should be varied and adapted to the shape of the liver.

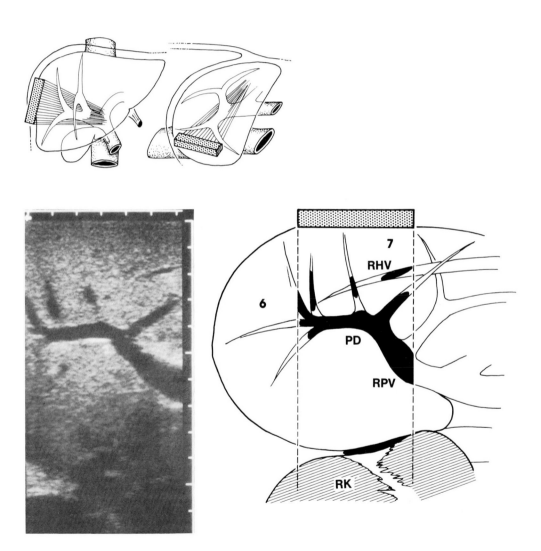

**Fig. 22.** The posterior division *(PD)* of the right portal vein *(RPV)* divides into two groups of smaller branches; those coursing superiorly (segment 7) are usually two or three in number, while three or four inferior branches perfuse segment 6. The right kidney is seen posteriorly *(RK)*. *RHV,* right hepatic vein. Posterior coronal section

# Tumors

Operative ultrasound permits the identification of hepatic tumors and their precise localization. The extent of spread and the presence of other lesions is determined, thus permitting proper planning of the surgical approach.

## Ultrasound Signs of Hepatic Tumors

The following ultrasound charateristics permit the identification of tumors [3]:

Variations in the echogenicity: the tumor can be hyper-, hypo-, or anechoic when compared to the surrounding hepatic parenchyma.
Tumors may be either homogeneous or heterogeneous.
The nature of the ultrasound beam beyond the lesion; it may be attenuated, increased, unchanged, or completely absent, i.e., an acoustic shadow.

*Anechoic Tumors.* The simple biliary cyst is the best example: it is round and completely anechoic with a thin, regular wall and posterior intensification of echoes (Fig. 23). Hydatid cysts are often sonolucent lesions presenting as a single liquid-filled space with a well-defined capsule (Fig. 24). They can also contain multiple liquid-filled compartments, which are the daughter cysts. The wall can be quite thick and will reflect echoes sharply if a significant degree of calcification is present. Operative ultrasound will detect communication with the biliary tree, which is often present. This finding has considerable therapeutic importance and will be discussed later in detail (see p. 54).

*Hyperechoic Tumors.* Hyperechoic tumors are of the following types. They are most commonly benign tumors such as angiomas (Fig. 25). Gastrointestinal tract metastases [14] (Fig. 26) are the second most common type in this group, and hepatocellular carcinomas present less frequently as hyperechoic lesions [8, 21].

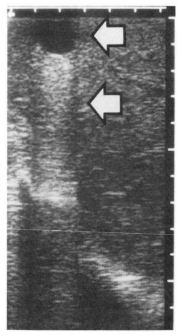

**Fig. 23.** Sonolucent lesion. A simple biliary cyst is shown; it is completely sonolucent with a thin regular wall *(upper arrow)* and posterior intensification of echoes *(lower arrow)*

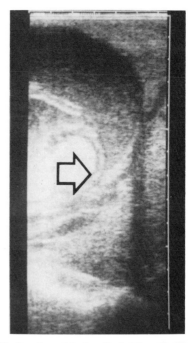

**Fig. 24.** Sonolucent lesion (hydatid cyst). The contents of the cyst are liquid, and there is septation of the interior and detachment of the wall *(arrow)*

*Hypoechoic Tumors.* Hypoechoic tumors are usually malignant, and are either metastatic lesions of extra-abdominal origin or primary hepatocellular carcinomas. Benign lesions are seen, but are less frequent. Hepatocellular carcinomas are often heterogeneous and locally extensive, with thrombosis of the portal vein branch draining the region. These tumors are often difficult to visualize, as they occur preferentially in cirrhotic livers which produce a markedly heterogeneous image on ultrasound examination (Fig. 27). Small lesions tend to have well-defined margins and are usually easier to identify (Fig. 28).

Homogeneous lesions with a density approximating that of the surrounding hepatic parenchyma can be identified only by their mass effect on neighboring vascular structures (Fig. 29).

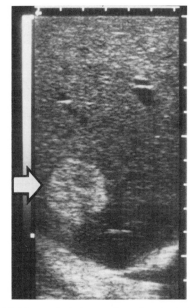

**Fig. 26.** Hyperechoic tumor: hepatic metastasis from an endocrine pancreatic tumor. The lesion is large (3 cm in diameter) and heterogeneous, with a surrounding halo *(arrow)*

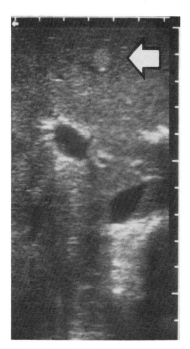

**Fig. 25.** Hyperechoic tumor: hemangioma. The lesion is homogeneous, hyperechoic, round, and well-demarcated. It is also small (8 mm; *arrow*)

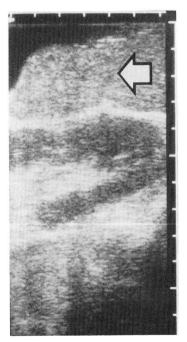

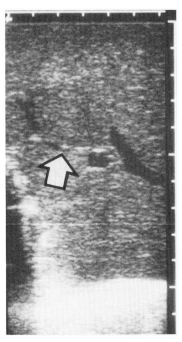

**Fig. 27.** Isoechoic tumor: hepatocellular carcinoma in a cirrhotic liver. The tumor *(arrow)* appears as a heterogeneous zone of about the same echogenicity as the surrounding parenchyma. A halo defining the limits of the tumor is seen

**Fig. 29.** Isoechoic tumor: hepatocellular carcinoma in cirrhosis. The tumor has nearly the same echodensity as the surrounding parenchyma, but is appreciated because of its mass effect: displacement of the hepatic vein branch *(arrow)*

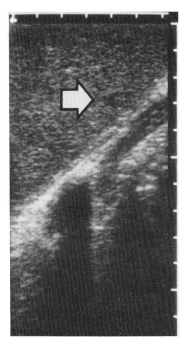

◄ **Fig. 28.** Hypoechoic tumor: hepatocellular carcinoma in a cirrhotic liver. This is a 7-mm tumor with a well-defined border *(arrow)*

## General Technique of Exploration

*Localization of the Tumor.* Diagnostic features are of greater importance in the preoperative ultrasound study than intraoperatively. In most cases ultrasound and other morphological examinations [angiography and computed tomography (CT) scanning] or biological tumor markers [alpha-fetoprotein, carcinoembryonic antigen (CEA)] permit a preoperative diagnosis and establish firmly the indication for surgery [12].

The role of operative ultrasound is to precisely localize the tumor. A meticulous study is done, and each abnormal finding is evaluated by altering the gain. It may be necessary to use the water pouch or to move the probe to the opposite side of the liver in order not to miss superficial lesions.

*Anatomical Study of the Liver.* The hepatic architecture should be studied completely to identify any anomalies which might be present. The identification of the hepatic veins and the portal pedicles is extremely useful in resectional surgery.

*Localization of the Tumor by Its Anatomical Relation to Other Structures.* The tumor may invade or displace major vascular structures. These findings will alter operative strategy and should be clarified before proceeding with resection [15].

For a small tumor in the right lobe, the relationship to the right hepatic vein and the segmental portal branches can be used to plan a limited anatomical resection. In major hepatic resection the position of the tumor in relation to the middle hepatic vein will determine the extent of resection (Figs. 30 and 31).

Vascular relationships are of key importance in determining resectability. A large tumor which by palpation seems localized to the right lobe can be determined by ultrasound to involve the left hepatic vein and thus be unresectable (Fig. 32). Central lesions can involve the hilus or compress a major portal branch or the vena cava.

Operative ultrasound can address these precise anatomical relationships more accurately than preoperative morphological examinations. Many different cross sections are studied to localize the lesion with respect to surface landmarks, which will permit accurate transection of the liver parenchyma.

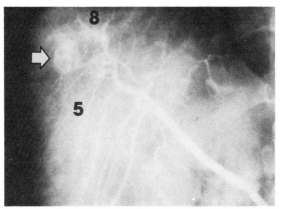 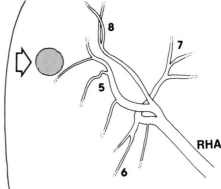

**Fig. 30 A**

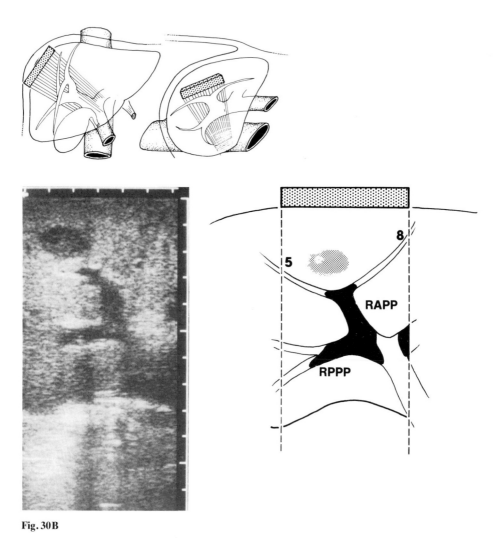

**Fig. 30 B**

**Fig. 30 A, B.** A 42-year-old man, followed up for 4 years because of postnecrotic cirrhosis, underwent ultrasound examination because of a slight elevation of alpha-fetoprotein (35 ng/ml with a normal level of less than 6). A hypoechoic lesion was identified which could not be localized precisely. **A** Arteriogram revealed that the lesion *(arrow)* was supplied by the right hepatic artery *(RHA)* and was located between segments 5 and 8. Intraoperatively, no lesion could be appreciated in the cirrhotic parenchyma by palpation of the liver. **B** Ultrasound was then performed, and localized the lesion to segment 8, making a limited resection possible. *RAPP,* anterior right portal pedicle; *RPPP,* posterior right portal pedicle

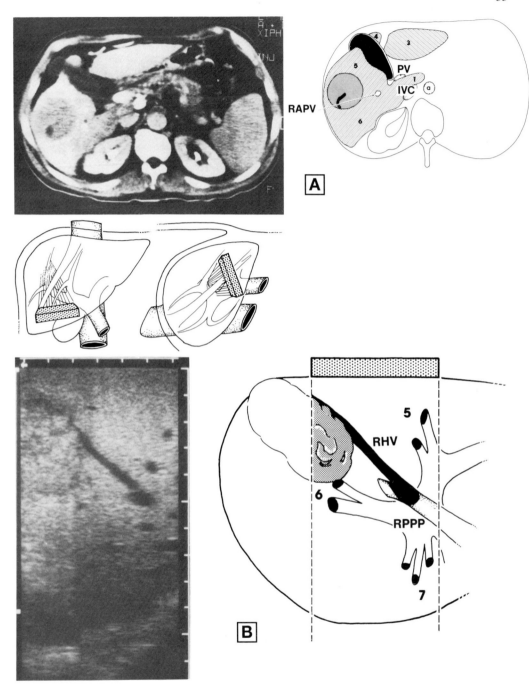

**Fig. 31A, B.** This 63-year-old man had a liver metastasis which was discovered by a screening ultrasound examination 6 months after abdominoperineal resection for adenocarcinoma of the rectum. **A** By CT scan the lesion appears to be located between segments 5 and 6. *a,* aorta; *PV,* portal vein; *IVC,* inferior vena cava; *RAPV,* anterior right portal vein. **B** Operative ultrasound showed that the lesion was located in segment 6 with invasion of the right hepatic vein *(RHV)* and segment 5; the patient treated by bisegmentectomy of 5 and 6. *RPPP,* posterior right portal pedicle

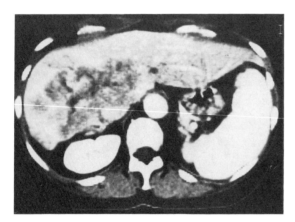

**Fig. 32A**

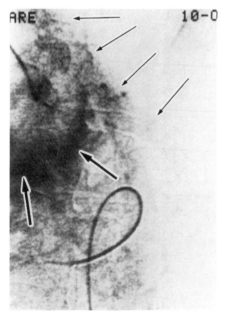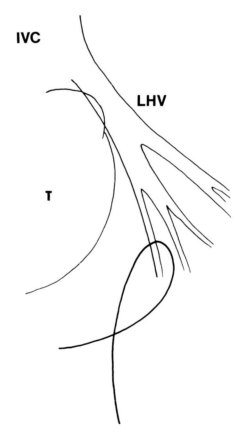

**Fig. 32B**

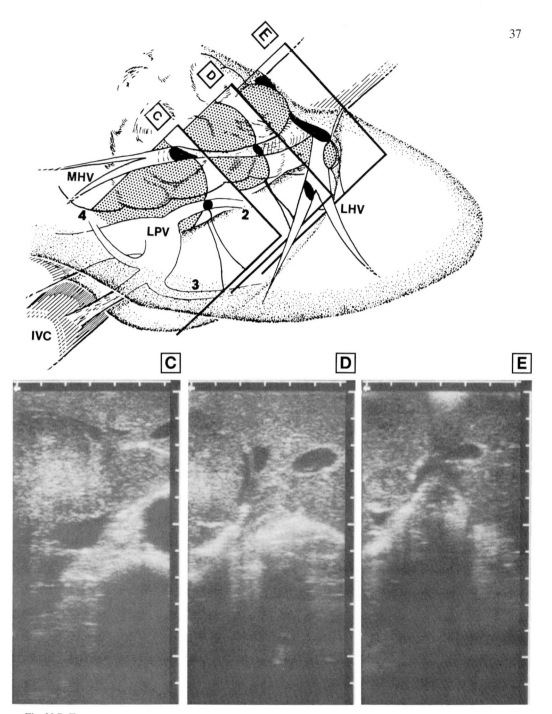

**Fig. 32 C–E**

**Fig. 32 A–E.** This 45-year-old woman presented with a large hepatic metastasis from an endocrine tumor of the pancreas. Preoperative studies, especially **A** CT scan, suggested that the lesion was confined to the right lobe. **B** Digital subtraction angiography suggested that the left hepatic vein *(LHV, thin arrows)* was patent, and that the tumors *(thick arrows)* were confined to the right lobe. **C, D, E** Operative ultrasound demonstrates extension of the tumor into the caudate lobe with posterior encasement of the left hepatic vein, making resection impossible. *MHV,* middle hepatic vein; *LPV,* left portal vein

*Evaluation of Tumor Extension.* Operative ultrasound permits the identification of primary or metastatic tumors which were unsuspected preoperatively. Such lesions are usually less than 2.5 cm in diameter.

The results of a prospective study of imaging in 34 patients with hepatic tumors are summarized in Table 1. Of these, 32 patients had arteriograms, all patients had preoperative ultrasound performed by the same examiner, and all patients had operative ultrasound. For lesions less then 1 cm in diameter, operative ultrasound is clearly much more sensitive. In this regard, the intraoperative discovery of a small tumor in the contralateral lobe would make it possible to avoid major hepatic resection in a patient who would not benefit from the procedure.

*Biopsy of Lesions with Ultrasound.* Histologic confirmation must be obtained by biopsy. This may require some mobilization of the liver to permit safe access to the lesion. A 19-gauge Menghini needle is used, as it is of large caliber and provides an adequate specimen. The tract of the needle is passed through normal parenchyma to permit control of hemorrhage from the procedure. To reduce the risk of dissemination, the trajectory should be planned so that it will be confined within the particular specimen which might require resection.

A guide fixed at a predetermined angle is attached to the ultrasound probe. The biopsy needle is advanced under ultrasound guidance. The point of the biopsy needle should be abraded to maximize the diffraction of the ultrasound beam and thus permit exact visualization of the point of the needle (Fig. 33).

**Modification of Surgical Tactics**

The use of operative ultrasound has modified our surgical approach to hepatic tumors.

At exploration, a limited incision is made initially to permit manual exploration of the abdominal cavity and ultrasound examination of the liver. If no obvious contraindication to resection is identified, the incision is then enlarged to complete the exploration, the liver is mobilized, and any biopsies which are necessary are performed before proceeding with resection.

*Surgical Treatment of Hepatocellular Carcinoma in Cirrhosis.* Modification of the hepatic parenchyma in cirrhosis often prevents the localization of hepatic tumors by palpation. The use of ultrasound thus becomes extremely important.

The "portal factor" plays a predominant role in these lesions, since the intrahepatic dissemination of these tumors is thought to occur via the portal venous system (Fig. 34) [7, 19]. Intrahepatic portal branches show tumor invasion upstream in 60%–70% of hepatocellular carcinomas [18]. Less commonly, thrombosis is observed in the hepatic

**Table 1.** Results of a prospective study of the imaging of hepatic tumors, comparing selective arteriography and pre- and intraoperative ultrasound[a]

| Diagnostic modality | Total nodules identified | Nodules less than 25 mm in diameter | Nodules less than 10 mm in diameter |
|---|---|---|---|
| Selective arteriography | 35%–51% | 5%–29% | 1%– 4% |
| Preoperative ultrasound | 55%–69% | 14%–82% | 4%–15% |
| Operative ultrasound | 65%–81% | 15%–88% | 13%–50% |

[a] A total of 80 lesions were evaluated from 16 patients with liver metastases, 15 patients with primary hepatocarcinomas, and 3 patients with benign lesions.

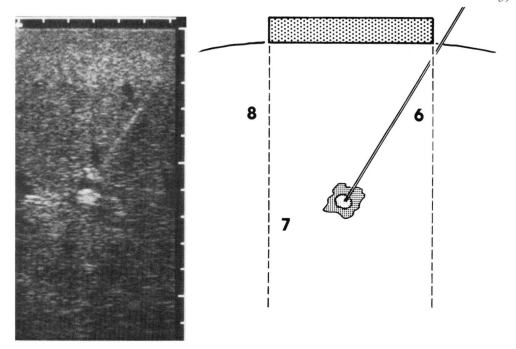

**Fig. 33.** This 48-year-old man had a single large liver metastasis in segment *3* identified by a preoperative ultrasound examination which was done to evaluate an elevation of the CEA level. Operative ultrasound showed another, hyperechoic lesion 8 mm in diameter surrounded by a hypoechoic halo; biopsy with frozen section determined it to be a metastasis in segment *7*

venous system. Neoplastic portal thrombosis propagates retrogradely toward the main portal venous trunk. At each portal bifurcation, tumor emboli then flow peripherally to establish a pattern of intrahepatic metastasis based on the portal system [13]. Adequate resectional surgery must thus encompass the entire hepatic region distal to the portal thrombosis. These considerations are of paramount importance in the cirrhotic liver, where the amount of resected hepatic parenchyma is related to the risk of the development of postoperative hepatic insufficiency. The extent of resection determined by the portal thrombosis does not always correspond to the classic segmental anatomy of Couinaud, but can be delineated by operative ultrasound.

Neoplastic portal venous thrombi appear as echogenic densities within the lumen of the vessel, which is normally an echo-free space, surrounded by Glisson's capsule (Figs. 35 and 36). The most distal portal bifurcation which is free of tumor can thus be identified and biopsied to establish the margin of resection (Fig. 37). In addition, using arteriographic techniques, a balloon catheter can be advanced under ultrasound guidance into the appropriate portal branch and distal flow thus be occluded. This portal occlusion can facilitate the parenchymal dissection which is more difficult in the cirrhotic patient (Fig. 38). The relevant arterial branch can be cannulated after hilar dissection and injected with methylene blue to mark the limits of resection. Using such techniques, the surgical treatment of hepatocellular carcinoma is based on precise anatomical and oncological information [2, 10].

Resective surgery remains the only treatment which can offer a chance of cure in this disease. Recent reports from Japanese [11],

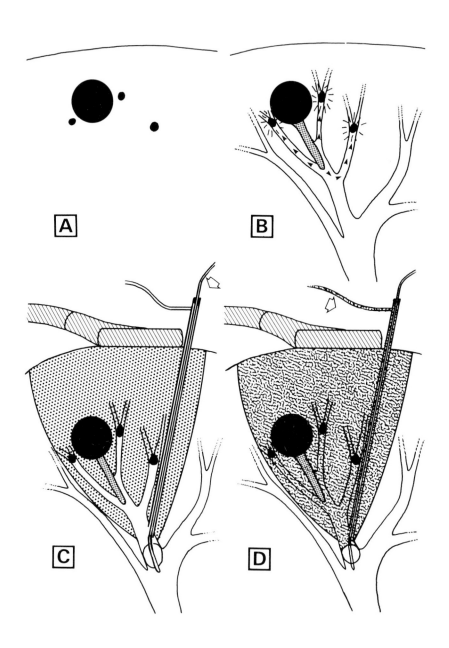

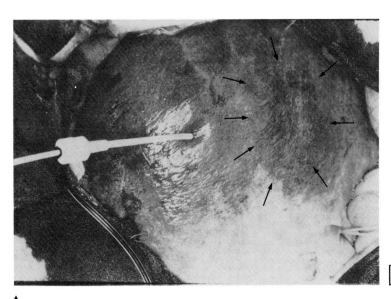

E

▲

◄ **Fig. 34A–E.** Adjustment in surgical tactics due to operative ultrasound of hepatic carcinoma. **A** The "classic" notion of metastatic spread shows the primary tumor surrounded by daughter lesions. **B** Portal propagation of tumor by thrombosis which progresses proximally, distributing neoplastic emboli distally at each portal bifurcation. **C** Using an introducer system, a balloon catheter *(arrow)* is guided into the portal system to perform an elective occlusion. **D** The catheter can also be used to inject a dye *(arrow)*, which will mark the parenchyma at risk from portal embolization and tumor spread. **E** Photograph showing the catheter in place with the coloration of the liver surface corresponding to the defined portal territory *(arrows)*

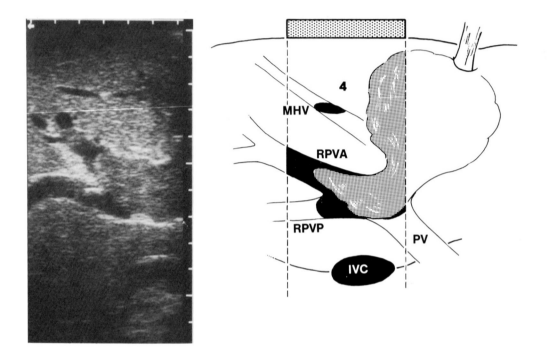

**Fig. 35.** This 55-year-old man with alcoholic cirrhosis developed a hepatocellular carcinoma of segments *3* and *4*. Preoperatively, ultrasound showed a lesion in segment *4* with portal thrombosis limited to the left portal vein branch. Intraoperatively, ultrasound showed that the thrombus extended beyond the bifurcation to the right portal vein branch, though it did not appear to be adherent to the vessel walls. Left hepatectomy with removal of the right portal thrombus was performed. *MHV*, middle hepatic vein; *RPVP*, posterior branch of the right portal vein; *RPVA*, anterior branch of the right portal vein; *IVC*, inferior vena cava; *PV*, portal vein

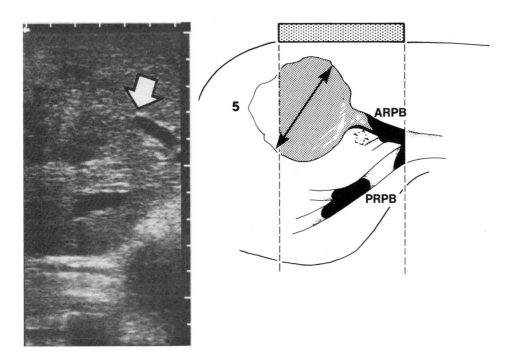

**Fig. 36.** A hepatocellular carcinoma of segment 5 *(white arrow)* was seen on preoperative ultrasound examination in a 58-year-old man with alcoholic cirrhosis. Intraoperatively it was possible to localize the tumor (a 4.5-cm lesion between the *black arrows*) with relation to the bifurcation of the right portal vein. *ARPB*, anterior right portal branch; *PRPB*, posterior right portal branch. The origin of the segmental branch to 5 is visible (5 mm in diameter) and it contains a 1-cm segment of thrombus *(dotted arrow)*

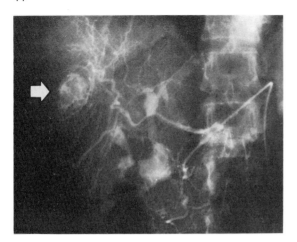

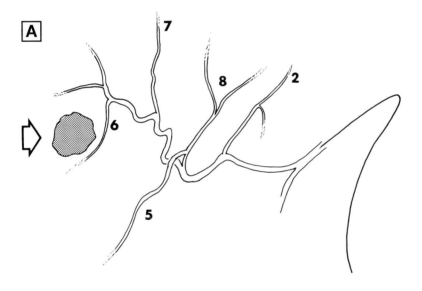

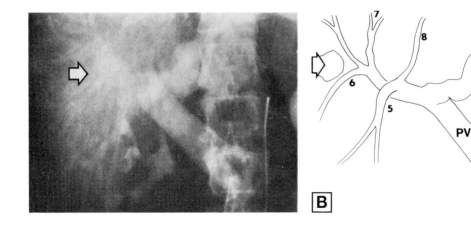

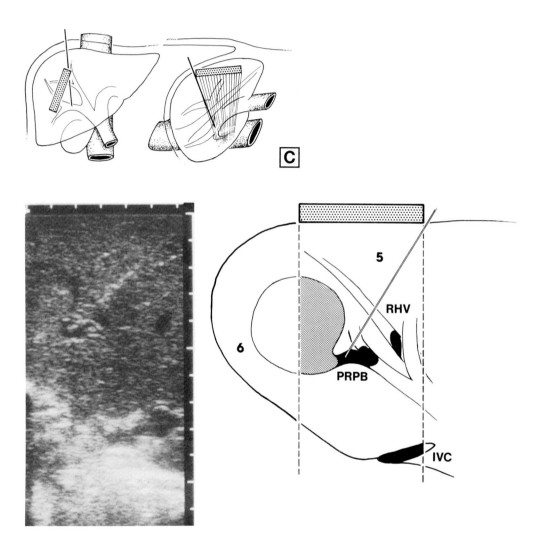

◄ **Fig. 37A–C.** This 55-year-old man with postnecrotic cirrhosis had a hepatocarcinoma of segment 6 identified by a routine ultrasound examination. Alpha-fetoprotein was normal. Arteriogram localized the tumor to segment 6 (**A**) and showed no portal thrombosis in the venous phase (**B**). Intraoperatively, ultrasound showed portal thrombosis of the branch feeding the tumor (**C**). This was punctured under ultrasound guidance and opacified with contrast to delineate the portal territory distal to the thrombus. *RHV*, right hepatic vein; *PRPB*, posterior right portal branch; *IVC*, inferior vena cava; *PV*, portal vein

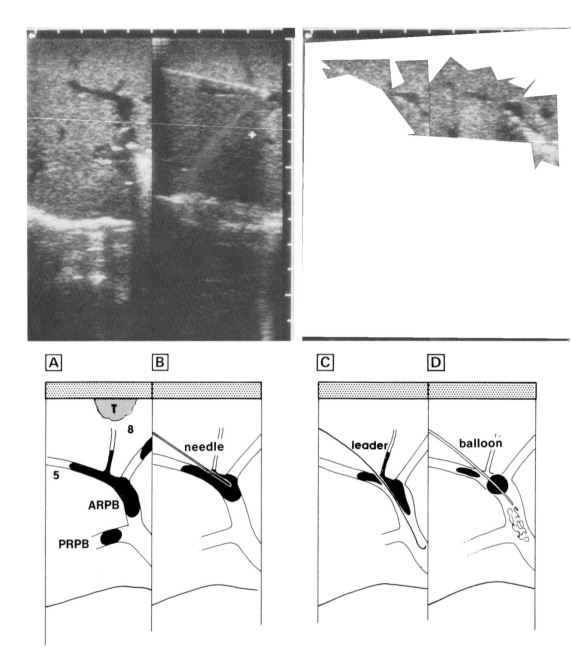

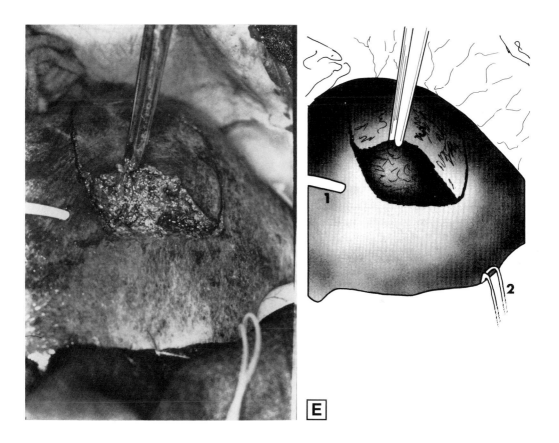

▲

◄ **Fig. 38 A–E.** This 62-year-old man with cirrhosis presented with a hepatocellular carcinoma, which was pre-operatively localized to segment *8* by arteriography and ultrasound. Intraoperatively, the tumor, which measured 2 cm in diameter, was found in the right portion of segment *8*. **A** Localization of the portal vein branch feeding the tumor (I). *ARPB,* anterior right portal branch; *PRPB,* posterior right portal branch. **B** Puncture of the branch with an 18-gauge needle *(above, white cross; below, needle).* **C** Insertion of a guidewire *(leader)* to permit placement of an introducer. **D** Positioning of a balloon catheter by injecting a small amount of saline containing air microbubbles. The balloon is then inflated to occlude the appropriate portal bifurcation. **E** Intra-operative photograph and diagram of the catheter and the introducer in place in the portal vein *(1)*. A Silastic loop has also been placed around the hepatic artery *(2)*. Vascular occlusion will then produce a demarcation of the territory to be resected *(3)* and permit a bloodless dissection

48

and Chinese [22] centers indicate that 5-year survivals exceeding 50% can be achieved in the treatment of small hepatocarcinomas.

Embolization of the portal branch of the tumor under ultrasound control can be performed as a palliative treatment in cases where resection is not possible (Fig. 39). The propagation of portal vein thrombosis can also be controlled to prevent the complica-tions of portal hypertension and variceal bleeding. Intermittent occlusion of the hepa-tic artery is useful in palliation, as it produces tumor ischemia and may enhance the efficacy of chemotherapy. The technique involves the placement of Silastic loops around the hepa-tic arterial branch perfusing the tumor, which are then used postoperatively to occlude flow to the tumor.

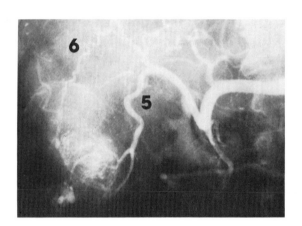

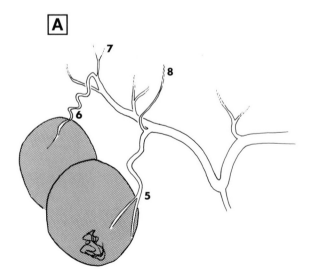

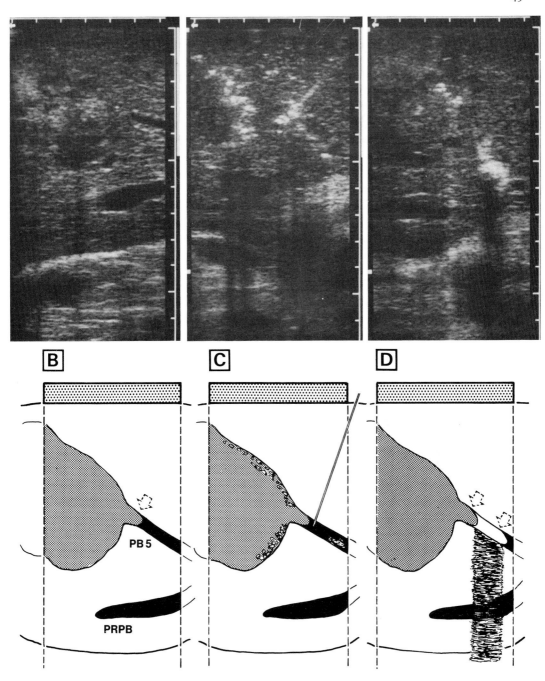

▲
◀ **Fig. 39 A–D.** This 62-year-old man with Laennec's cirrhosis had a hepatocellular carcinoma of segments 5 and 6 documented by arteriography (**A**). At surgery, peritoneal carcinomatosis was present contraindicating resection. **B** By ultrasound guidance the portal branch *(PB5)* supplying the tumor, which contained a thrombus *(dotted arrows),* was punctured *PRPB,* posterior right portal branch. **C** The position of the needle was confirmed by injecting a small amount of saline containing air microbubbles. **D** Embolization *(dotted arrows)* of the tumor was then carried out using bucrylate, which produces marked acoustic shadows

*Second-Look Operations.* In our patients systematic reexploration is performed 1 year after the initial treatment to rule out recurrence in patients who are doing well. Operative ultrasound is important in these procedures, because it permits the detection of small lesions which are difficult to palpate in the hypertrophied remnant liver. In addition, postoperative changes and hypertrophy make precise localization of the lesions impossible by palpation. Ultrasound provides a clear definition of the vascular architecture with relation to the tumor, which is critical when performing secondary resections (Fig. 40).

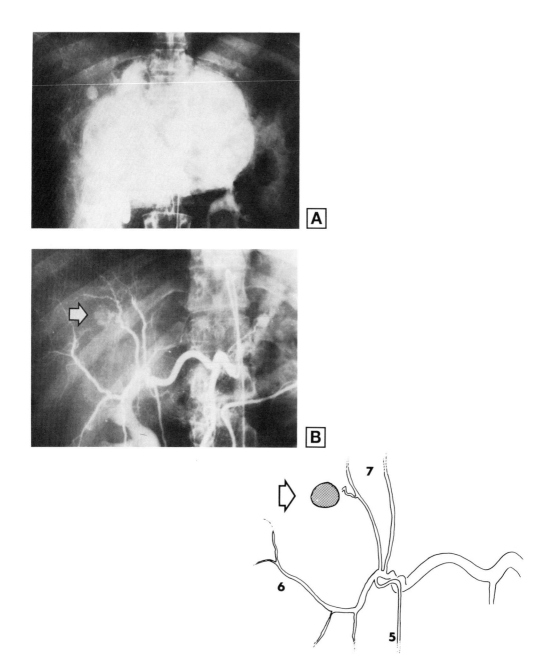

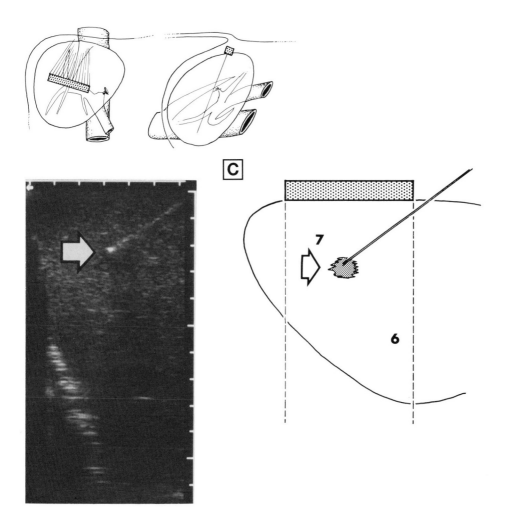

▲
◀ **Fig. 40A–C.** A large hepatocellular carcinoma was found in a 28-year-old pregnant woman. **A** The lesion was in the left lobe and associated with a normal alpha-fetoprotein level. The patient was treated nonoperatively for 1 year with chemotherapy and two successive percutaneous embolizations. She then underwent left hepatectomy extended to include segment 8. Postoperatively she received further chemotherapy. **B** The patient underwent reexploration 1 year later, at which time arteriography showed a 1-cm hypervascular lesion *(arrow)*. **C** The lesion was not palpable at surgery, despite complete mobilization of the liver. Using ultrasound, the lesion was punctured with a Menghini needle *(arrow)*. A frozen section was positive for tumor. Segmental resection was performed, and the patient is now well 18 months later, with no evidence of recurrence

52

*Surgical Therapy of Metastatic Tumors.* Detection of small nodules is critical in the therapy of metastatic disease. By precise localization of the lesion with respect to the portal pedicles, formal segmental resections can be performed [2] (Fig. 41). These have a lower operative risk than major hepatectomies and also permit subsequent resections if necessary. Formal segmental resections probably have a better prognosis than simple metastasectomy [1]. During these procedures, blood loss can be reduced by the intraluminal placement of a balloon catheter to occlude the portal branch during resection.

In small inaccessible central lesions, palliative treatment can consist of transhepatic electrocoagulation of the tumor. Using a Teflon-coated needle under ultrasound guidance, the coagulation is performed directly, without injury to the surrounding hepatic parenchyma (Fig. 42).

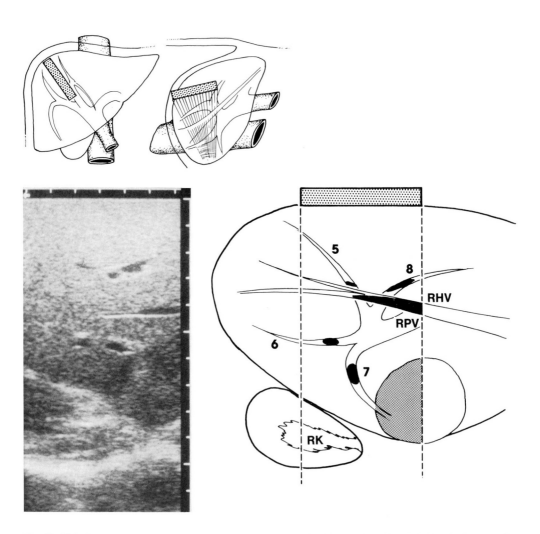

**Fig. 41.** This 62-year-old woman presented with a liver metastasis 6 months after right hemicolectomy for adenocarcinoma. A solitary lesion in segment 7 was localized by operative ultrasound and resection was performed. *RPV,* right portal vein; *RHV,* right hepatic vein; *RK,* right kidney

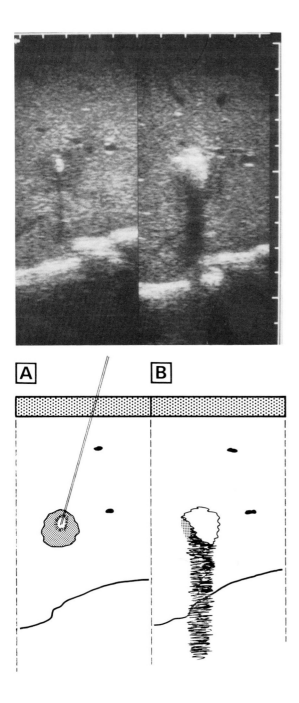

**Fig. 42 A, B.** This 61-year-old man presented with a large metastasis in the right lobe, which was treated by right hepatectomy. At exploration a small lesion in segment *4* was found, which was treated by electrocoagulation. **A** Puncture of the nodule under ultrasound guidance. The point of the needle is very echogenic and is clearly visible in this study. **B** Electrocoagulation results in modification of the ultrasound properties of the tumor, which becomes very hyperechoic

## Operative Ultrasound in the Surgery of Hydatid Cysts

Since the diagnosis in this disease is usually established preoperatively, operative ultrasound is primarily useful in planning therapy. On ultrasound examination, the cyst appears as an area of liquid density with posterior intensification of the echoes. When daughter cysts are present, they produce a honeycomb pattern within the cyst. Calcification is also a frequent finding, and it produces intense echogenicity.

Operative ultrasound has three main applications in the treatment of hydatid cystes:

1. The establishment of the relationship of the cyst to major vascular structures

2. The identification of biliary fistulas (Fig. 43)

3. Examination of the hepatic parenchyma and the biliary tree for the presence of daughter cysts, which can lead to complications of biliary obstruction and recurrence of the disease (Fig. 44)

## Operative Ultrasound in the Treatment of Pyogenic Liver Abscesses

Operative therapy of these lesions becomes necessary if percutaneous drainage [20] has been unsuccessful. During surgery ultrasound [9] is used to identify loculations and secondary collections, as well as to guide the proper placement of the drains (Fig. 45).

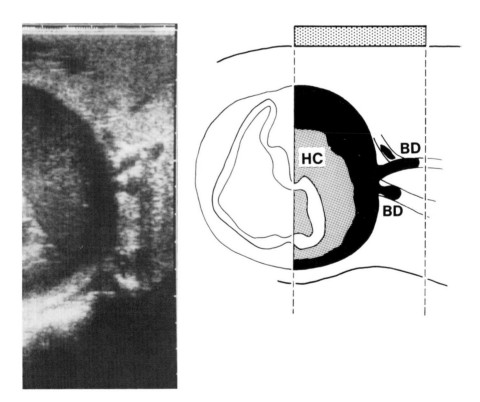

**Fig. 43.** This 24-year-old woman presented with a large hydatid cyst *(HC)* in the right liver. Operative ultrasound revealed a double biliary fistula, which was found when the cyst was opened. *BD,* bile duct of segment *8*

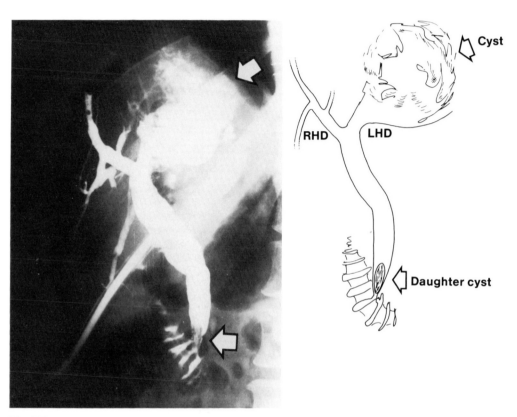

Fig. 44 A

56

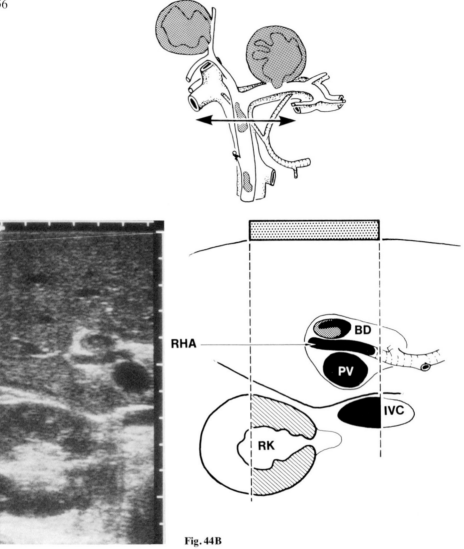

Fig. 44B

**Fig. 44 A, B.** This 42-year-old man had been previously treated for cholangitis with the placement of a T-tube. He had two large hydatid cysts of segment *1*. **A** T-tube cholangiogram shows the communication between the left hepatic duct *(LHD)* and the *cyst* in segment *1*. At least one *daughter cyst* is seen in the distal common bile duct *(RHD,* right hepatic duct). **B** This finding is confirmed by operative ultrasound, which clearly shows the daughter cyst in the common bile duct *(BD)*. *RHA,* right branch of hepatic artery; *PV,* portal vein; *IVC,* inferior vena cava; *RK,* right kidney

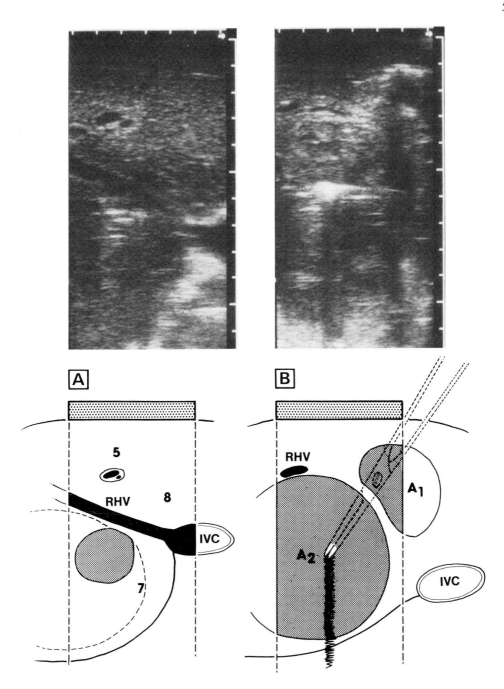

**Fig. 45A, B.** This 43-year-old man had a pyogenic liver abscess of segment 7. He did not respond to antibiotics and percutaneous drainage. **A** At surgery ultrasound permits the localization of the abscess with respect to the right hepatic vein *(RHV). IVC,* inferior vena cava. **B** Several loculations were present *(A1, A2);* these were identified and disrupted. Ultrasound was useful in assuring proper placement of the drains

58

# References

1. Adson MA, Van Heerden VA (1980) Major hepatic resections for metastatic colorectal cancer. Ann Surg 191:576–583
2. Bismuth H, Houssin D, Castaing D (1982) Major and minor segmentectomies "réglées" in liver surgery. World J Surg 6:10–24
3. Bruneton TN, Dageville X, Fenalt D, et al (1982) Les masses hépatiques en échographie: à propos de 400 cas. J Radiol 63:181–187
4. Chafetz N, Filly RA (1979) Portal hepatic veins: accuracy of margin echoes for distinguishing intra hepatic vessels. Radiology 130:725–728
5. Couinaud C (1957) Le foie: études anatomiques et chirurgicales. Masson, Paris
6. Duvauferrier R, Duvauferrier-Pellenc MC, Simon J, et al (1980) Anatomie échographique du foie. Ultrasonics 1:113–119
7. Edmonson HA (1958) Tumors of the liver and intrahepatic bile ducts. Force institute of pathology, Washington 32:109
8. Freeny PC, Vimont TR, Barnett DC (1979) Cavernous hemangioma of the liver: ultrasonography, arteriography and computed tomography. Radiology 132:143–148
9. Glen PM, Noseworthy J, Babcock DS (1984) Use of intra-operative ultrasonography to localize a hepatic abscess. Arch Surg 119:347–348
10. Hasegawa H, Shimamura S (1984) Communication aus XXII$^{eme}$ Journées de Chirurgie hépato-biliaire, Paris
11. Kanematsu T, Takenaka K, Matsumata T, et al (1984) Limited hepatic resection for selected cirrhotic patients with primary liver cancer. Ann Surg 199:51–56
12. Kitazawa E, Machit A, Aiso Y, et al (1983) An evaluation of ultrasound in detection of small hepatocellular carcinoma in comparison with alphafoetoprotein. Gastroenterology 3:1070
13. Kishi K, Shikata T, Hirohashi S, et al (1983) Hepatocellular carcinoma, a clinical and pathologic analysis of 57 hepatectomy cases. Cancer 51:542–548
14. Kunstlinger F (1983) Découverte échographique fortuite de lésions focalisées du foie. Gastroenterol Clin Biol 7:951–954
15. Makuuchi M, Hasegawa H, Yamazaki S (1981) Intraoperative ultrasonic examination for hepatectomy. Jap J Clin Oncol 11:367–389
16. Makuuchi M, Hasegawa H, Yamazaki S, et al (1983) The inferior right hepatic vein: ultrasonic demonstration. Radiology 148:213–217
17. Marks WM, Filly RA, Callen PW (1979) Ultrasonic anatomy of the liver: a review with new applications. J Clin Ultrasounds 7:137–146
18. Martin E, Feldmann G (1983) Histopathologie du foie et des voies biliaires. Masson, Paris, p 293
19. Nakashima T (1975) Vascular changes and hemodynamics in hepatocellular carcinoma. In: Okuda K, Peters RL (eds) Hepatocellular carcinoma. J Wiley, New York, pp 196–197
20. Roemer CE, Ferrucci JT, Mueller PR, et al (1981) Hepatic cysts: diagnosis and therapy by sonographic nnedle aspiration. Am J Roentgenol 136:1065–1070
21. Roger JV, Mack LA, Freeny PC, et al (1981) Hepatic focal nodular hyperplasia: angiography, CT, sonography and scintigraphy. Am J Radiol 137:983–990
22. Yu K, Tang Z, Zhou X (1980) Experience in resection of small hepatocellular carcinoma. Chin Med J 93:491–495

# 3 Operative Ultrasound in Biliary Surgery

The earliest application of operative ultrasound was in the study of the extrahepatic bile ducts. Since 1965 this technique has been advocated to complement cholangiography [4, 9]. A-mode ultrasound was used initially, but is difficult to perform and interpret. The introduction of B-mode real-time ultrasound with the work of Lane and Glazer [10] and Sigel et al. [12, 13] has made possible the wide application of operative ultrasound.

Multiple applications of operative ultrasound are possible in biliary surgery: in anatomical study, in the evaluation of cholelithiasis and choledocholithiasis, in intrahepatic stone disease, and in the study of biliary tract tumors.

## Anatomical Study

The anatomical study is best divided into three parts: the gallbladder and the extrahepatic and intrahepatic bile ducts. The technical demands of these studies are of varying degrees of difficulty (Fig. 46).

## Gallbladder

The gallbladder is usually easy to study, since the fundus is visible at the anterior edge of the liver. If the probe is placed on the anterior surface of the liver superiorly at the junction of segments 4 and 5, the gallbladder

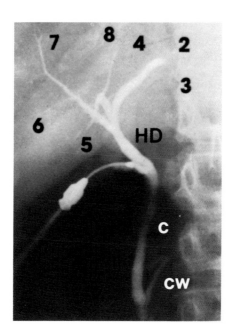
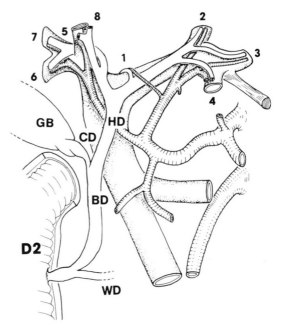

**Fig. 46.** Anatomy of the bile ducts seen by cholangiography. The right hepatic duct is formed by the union of an anterior branch from segments 5 and 8 and a posterior branch from segments 6 and 7. The left hepatic duct is longer; it receives three main branches from segments 2, 3 and 4, as well as two or three smaller branches from segment 1. The junction of the two ducts at the biliary confluence is anterior to the portal bifurcation. The common hepatic duct *(HD)* is thus formed, and receives the cystic duct *(CD)* from the gallbladder *(GB)* to form the common bile duct *(BD)*. The common bile duct ends in most cases as a common channel with Wirsung's duct *(WD)*, at the level of the papilla in the second portion of the duodenum *(D2)*

is transhepatically visible, and appears as a sonolucent zone which narrows toward the common duct, where Hartmann's pouch is seen. The wall is thin (1–2 mm), with an echodensity slightly greater than that of the hepatic parenchyma. The course of the cystic duct is often difficult to see because of its small size, tortuous course, and the obstruction of the lumen by the spiral valves (Fig. 47).

In the normal gallbladder the lumen is sonolucent with posterior accentuation of echoes. Sometimes, with high gain, small mobile echoes are seen which do not produce acoustic shadows. These are different from "sludge," and their exact nature is unknown (difference in bile density?) Microlithiasis (stones less than 3 mm in diameter) has a more heterogeneous appearance, and is characterized by rapid sedimentation.

## Intrahepatic Bile Ducts

The intrahepatic biliary tree is easily seen by transhepatic study. The bile ducts arborize within the portal pedicles with the corresponding portal venous and hepatic arterial branches. The bile ducts are much smaller in size than the portal venous branches and are approximately the size of the arterial branches, which are distinguished by their pulsations. Peripherally within the parenchyma, the biliary radicles are seen as thin channels devoid of echoes.

The segmental channels are usually visible and the main intrahepatic bile ducts can always be seen at their confluence, which is anterior and slightly inferior to the portal venous confluence (Fig. 48).

## Extrahepatic Bile Ducts

These can be studied (a) by transverse sections in the hepatoduodenal ligament and (b) longitudinal sections which permit the visualization of the entire extrahepatic bile duct along its main axis. Its course is slightly oblique toward the left, with a gentle concavity toward the right.

The highest part of the bile duct is seen transhepatically through the quadrate lobe. The distal bile duct is examined by using the water pouch. Gentle pressure is applied over the duodenum to collapse its lumen and thus permit visualization of the intrapancreatic portion of the common duct without the impediment of the duodenal air.

*The Hilus.* The biliary convergence is large and easily found by ultrasound (Fig. 49). The common hepatic duct is usually 4–5 mm in diameter and is located anteriorly and slightly to the right of the portal vein bifurcation.

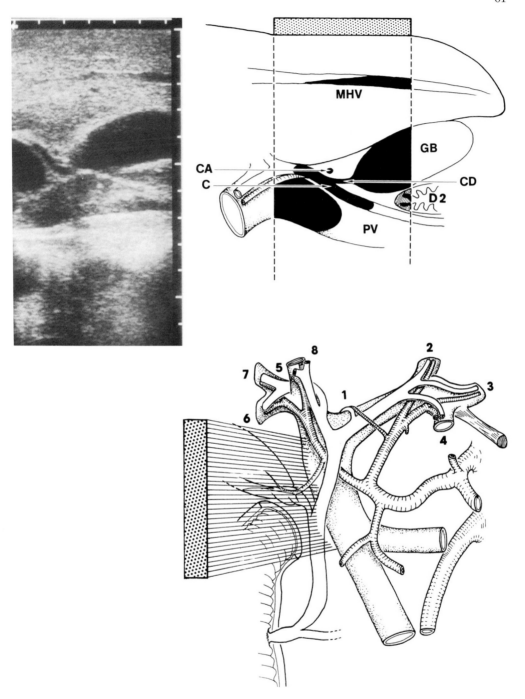

**Fig. 47.** The gallbladder *(GB)* and its neck empty into the cystic duct *(CD)*, which joins the common hepatic duct to form the common bile duct *(C)*. Intensification of echoes is seen posteriorly to the gallbladder. *CA,* cystic artery; *PV,* portal vein; *MHV,* middle hepatic vein; *D2,* second portion of the duodenum. Sagittal transhepatic section through gallbladder and hepatoduodenal ligament

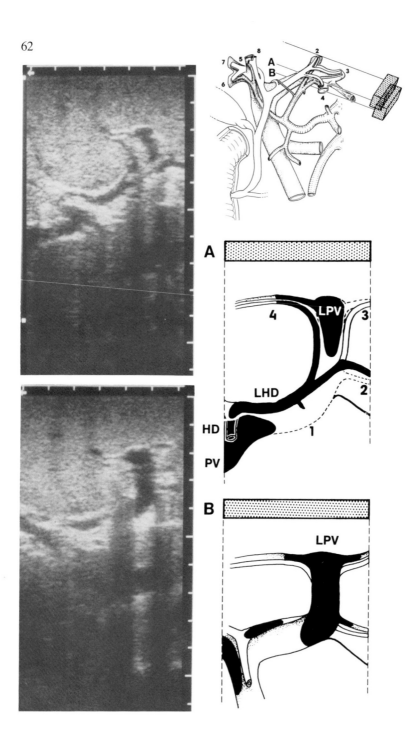

**Fig. 48A, B.** Left intrahepatic bile ducts. Section **A**, which is slightly superior to section **B**, shows the biliary convergence forming the common hepatic duct *(HD);* the left hepatic duct *(LHD)* is formed by the junction of segmental ducts *2, 3,* and *4.* A segmental duct of segment *1* measuring 1 mm in diameter is seen as it enters the left hepatic duct near the confluence. *LPV,* left branch of portal vein; *PV,* portal vein. Section **B** shows the left branch of the portal vein *(LPV)* in its anterior portion (recessus of Rex) as it divides into segmental branches for *2, 3,* and *4.* Horizontal transhepatic section to the left of the hilus near the anterior edge of the liver

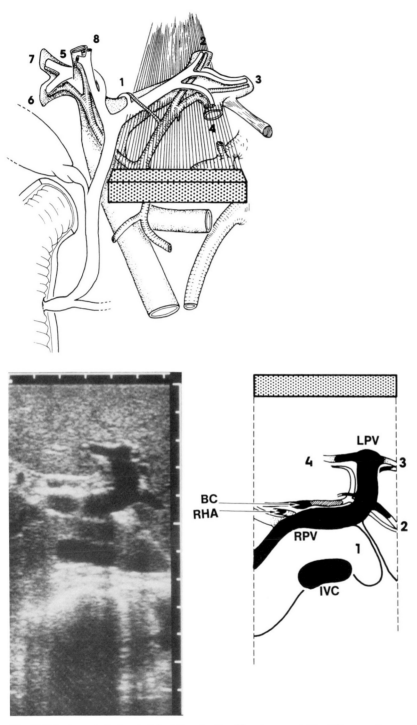

**Fig. 49.** Bile ducts at the level of the hilus visualized by ultrasound. The biliary confluence *(BC)* is anterior and slightly superior to the portal venous bifurcation. The right branch of the hepatic artery *(RHA)*, having crossed the plane of the common duct and the portal vein, remains to the right of the hepatoduodenal ligament. *IVC*, inferior vena cava; *LPV*, left portal vein branch; *RPV*, right portal vein branch. Horizontal transhepatic section through the hilus

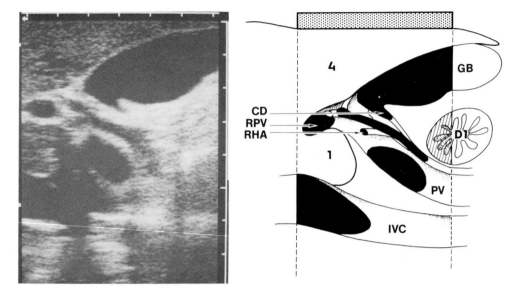

**Fig. 50.** The common hepatic duct is formed at the level of the hilus and is anterior to the portal vein. [Only the right portal vein *(RPV)* is visible in this section.] The right branch of the middle hepatic artery *(RHA)* passes between the common hepatic duct and the portal vein *(PV)*. It receives the cystic duct *(CD)* to form the common bile duct. *GB*, gallbladder; *IVC*, inferior vena cava; *D1*, first portion of the duodenum. Sagittal transhepatic section centered on the hepatoduodenal ligament and the gallbladder

*The Common Hepatic Duct.* The common hepatic duct (Fig. 50) is of constant diameter and is oriented vertically with a slight concavity to the right. As it courses distally it approaches the right border of the portal vein. At this level the right branch of the hepatic artery passes between the two, although it occasionally crosses anterior to the bile duct.

*The Common Bile Duct.* After receiving the cystic duct, the common bile duct (Fig. 51) separates from the portal vein and enters the pancreas behind the duodenum. At this point it deviates to the right to enter the second portion of the duodenum.

At the level of the pancreas its relations are with the portal vein and, to the left, the gastroduodenal artery with its pancreatoduodenal branches. To obtain the best anatomical study it is important to follow the entire course of each structure, beginning in the midportion of the hepatoduodenal ligament, where it is most easily identified.

*The Ampulla of Vater.* As the common bile duct is followed distally, it curves to the right through the pancreas. The pancreatic parenchyma is slightly more echogenic than the duodenal wall. If the duodenum is filled with air, it will block the ultrasound and produce a large acoustic shadow. Liquid contents will be anechoic. The junction of the common bile duct with Wirsung's duct is seen as a 2-mm channel (Fig. 52) with strongly echogenic walls. The papilla is best seen when there is little air in the duodenum, and appears as an excrescence protruding into the duodenal lumen.

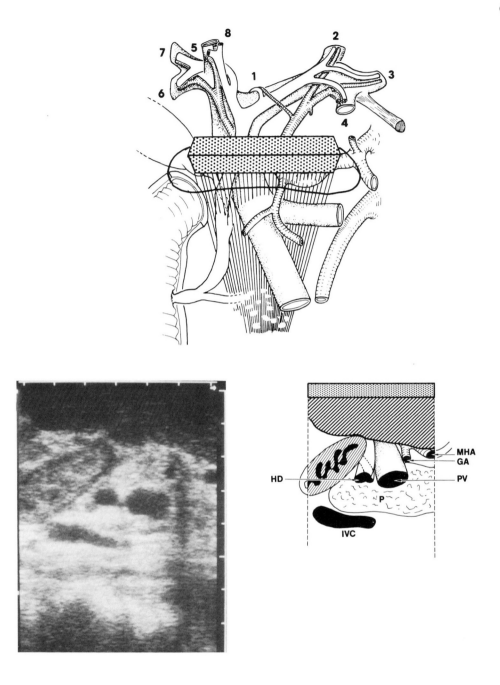

**Fig. 51.** Distal common bile duct. *MHA*, middle hepatic artery; *GA*, gastroduodenal artery; *PV*, portal vein; *HD*, common hepatic duct at its junction with the cystic duct; *P*, pancreas, with an echostructure which is more dense than that of the liver; *IVC*, inferior vena cava. Horizontal section using the water pouch *(hatched)* distally in the hepatoduodenal ligament

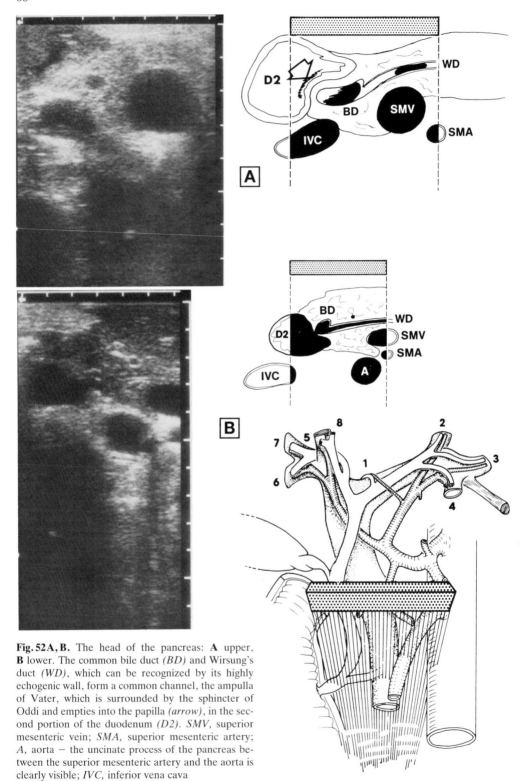

**Fig. 52 A, B.** The head of the pancreas: **A** upper, **B** lower. The common bile duct *(BD)* and Wirsung's duct *(WD)*, which can be recognized by its highly echogenic wall, form a common channel, the ampulla of Vater, which is surrounded by the sphincter of Oddi and empties into the papilla *(arrow)*, in the second portion of the duodenum *(D2)*. *SMV*, superior mesenteric vein; *SMA*, superior mesenteric artery; *A*, aorta − the uncinate process of the pancreas between the superior mesenteric artery and the aorta is clearly visible; *IVC*, inferior vena cava

# Cholelithiasis

Although the diagnosis of cholelithiasis is usually made preoperatively, operative ultrasound is useful in the following circumstances:

1. The detection of cholelithiasis in the patient who is being explored for another reason
2. The detection of microlithiasis

## Patients Undergoing Nonbiliary Abdominal Surgery

There is a considerable risk of postoperative cholecystitis in patients with cholelithiasis whose gallstones are not treated during abdominal surgery. The evaluation of the gallbladder is also important in the cirrhotic patient who is at increased risk of cholelithiasis [3] and tolerates complications poorly. Operative ultrasound is much more reliable than palpation in the diagnosis of cholelithiasis. Stones appear as highly echogenic, crescent-shaped structures in the sonolucent lumen of the gallbladder. They also produce a marked acoustic shadow (Figs. 53 and 54).

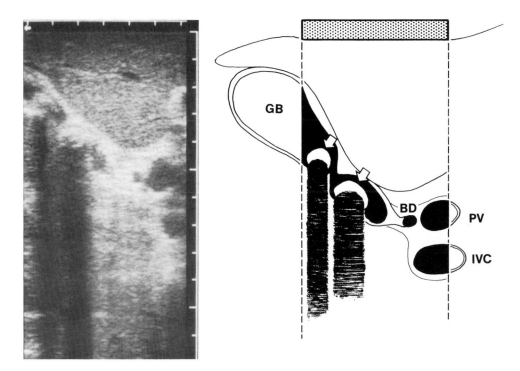

**Fig. 53.** This 51-year-old woman presented with a history of right upper quadrant pain suggestive of biliary colic, of several years' duration. Preoperative ultrasound demonstrated cholelithiasis. Operative ultrasound revealed calculi *(arrows)* and a thickened gallbladder *(GB)* wall, suggesting chronic cholelithiasis. The common bile duct *(BD)* is small and contains no calculi. This finding was confirmed by operative cholangiography. *PV,* portal vein; *IVC,* inferior vena cava. Horizontal section, slightly oblique, along the long axis of the gallbladder

### Microlithiasis of the Gallbladder

This can be a difficult diagnosis to establish using standard radiologic techniques. A high index of suspicion must be maintained in clinical situations such as recurrent subacute pancreatitis.

Microlithiasis (calculi less than 3 mm in diameter), is seen on ultrasound examination as small echogenic densities which do not produce acoustic shadows unless they coalesce (Fig. 55). They are different from sludge in that they are more echogenic, irregular, and sediment more rapidly with movement [1].

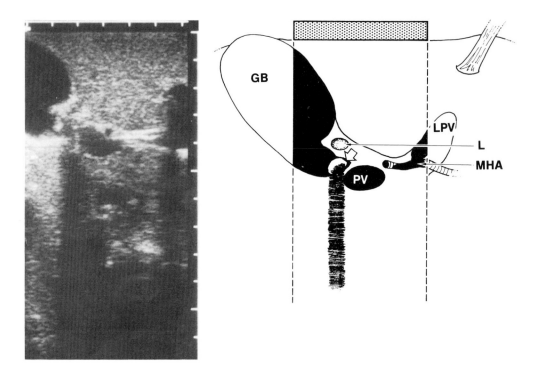

**Fig. 54.** This 36-year-old man presented with right upper quadrant pain with a palpable gallbladder *(GB)* on clinical examination. Ultrasound showed an enlarged gallbladder with homogeneous liquid content and thin walls. The common bile duct was normal. At surgery, hydrops of the gallbladder was found, with a stone *(arrow)* impacted in the gallbladder neck. These findings are seen on operative ultrasound. *PV,* portal vein; *MHA,* middle hepatic artery; *LPV,* left branch of portal vein; *L,* lymphadenopathy. Horizontal section, slightly oblique, through the long axis of the gallbladder

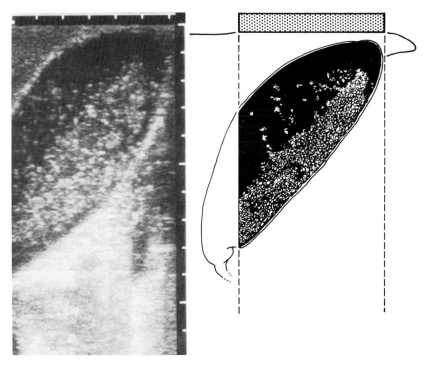

**Fig. 55.** This 43-year-old man presented with episodes of acute pancreatitis characterized by typical abdominal pain and marked amylasemia. Three previous episodes of pancreatitis had been documented. There was no history of alcohol abuse, and preoperative ultrasound and intravenous cholangiogram were normal. Intraoperatively the gallbladder was seen to be enlarged, with thin walls. Although no stones were palpated, ultrasound revealed the presence of multiple microcalculi, which were treated by cholecystectomy. Sagittal section along the long axis of the gallbladder

## Intrahepatic Lithiasis

Intrahepatic stone disease is defined as the presence of calculi in the portion of the biliary tree which is within the hepatic parenchyma. Lithiasis of the extrahepatic portion of the left hepatic duct is thus excluded from this category.

The following factors make this diagnosis difficult preoperatively:

Intravenous cholangiography rarely provides detail of the intrahepatic bile ducts adequate to identify small calculi.

More invasive procedures, such as percutaneous transhepatic cholangiography (PTC) or endoscopic retrograde cholangiography (ERC), are useful but carry some risk to the patient. They are not routinely indicated in intrahepatic lithiasis, and in addition may fail to identify small calculi proximal to a lesion.

Preoperative ultrasound is of value if a complete examination of the liver can be performed; however, evaluation in these patients is often limited by previous surgery or the morphology of the patient.

Because of these limitations, the diagnosis is often not made preoperatively. It can even be missed on the operative cholangiogram unless care is taken to fill the entire biliary tree (Fig. 56).

Operative ultrasound permits the identification of intrahepatic calculi as highly echogenic images within the ducts in the portal pedicles. Posteriorly they produce either an acoustic shadow or simple attenuation of the ultrasound beam. The calculus is usually associated with dilatation of the segmental bile duct (Fig. 57).

Diagnostic confusion can exist in the following instances:

1. Aerobilia (air bubbles in the bile) can produce echogenic images with acoustic shadows, especially when the bile duct is perpendicular to the ultrasound beam. This image is usually narrower than that produced by calculi, and varies rapidly in position as the liver is moved (Fig. 58). An additional problem is that the presence of aerobilia will mask small calculi which may be present.
2. Very distal portal pedicles with a small diameter can also produce an image suggestive of small calculi. The walls of these small structures are highly echogenic and the lumens are not visible.

Among 12 patients with intrahepatic lithiasis the diagnosis was made preoperatively in 9 by ultrasound. Of these patients, 7 also had operative ultrasound, which was diagnostic in 6 cases. The false-negative diagnoses arrived at by ultrasound were due to aerobilia in all cases but one, in which the findings were considered to be normal.

In addition to providing diagnostic and topographic information, operative ultrasound has therapeutic applications in this disease. To supplement the classic techniques of dealing with intrahepatic stones, ultrasound permits transhepatic maneuvers to deal with the problem from above the stricture. By advancing a needle and using a guidewire, a balloon catheter can be introduced into the distal biliary tree to dilate strictures by the Grüntzig technique [6]. In this way, previously inaccessible high strictures can be treated either by dilatation or by placement of drains which provide access for percutaneous manipulations postoperatively.

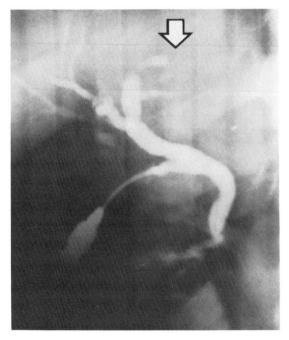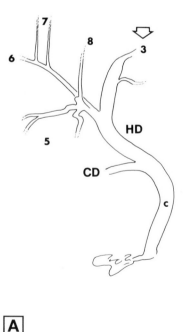

Fig. 56 A

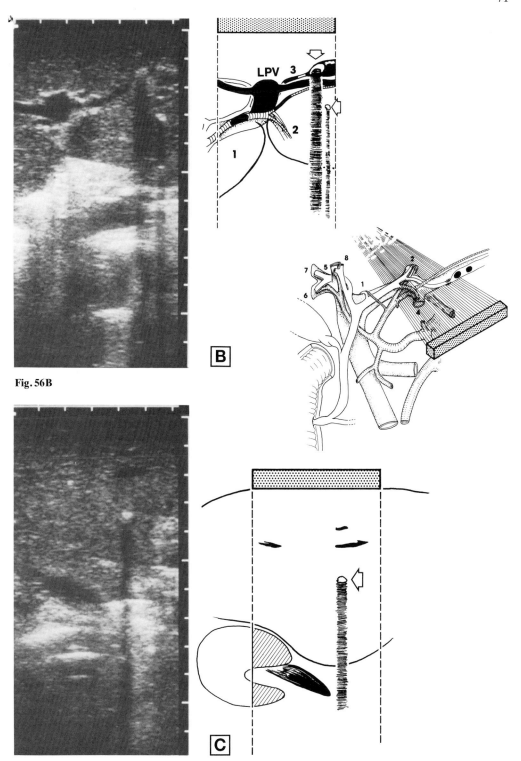

**Fig. 56 B**

**Fig. 56 C**

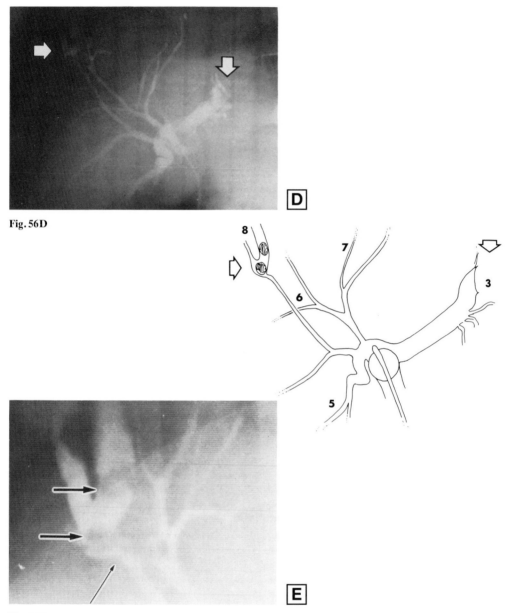

**Fig. 56D**

**Fig. 56E**

**Fig. 56A–E.** This 60-year-old man, who presented with an episode of acute pancreatitis, was found by intravenous cholangiography to have cholelithiasis. **A** Intraoperatively, radiomanometry, despite pressure to 28 cm $H_2O$, did not completely fill the left ductal system *(arrow)*. *c,* common bile duct; *HD,* common hepatic duct; *CD,* cystic duct. **B, C** Operative ultrasound demonstrated intrahepatic calculi *(arrows)* lodged in the ducts of segment (**B**; left liver) and segment *8* (**C**; right liver). These had not been suspected preoperatively. The common bile duct was normal. *LPV,* left branch of portal vein. A second cholangiogram was performed using a Foley catheter, which **D** showed the presence of calculi *(arrows)* and **E** demonstrated areas of stenosis *(thin arrow)* with proximal ductal dilatation *(broader arrows)*. Horizontal section through the round ligament at the anterior edge of the liver

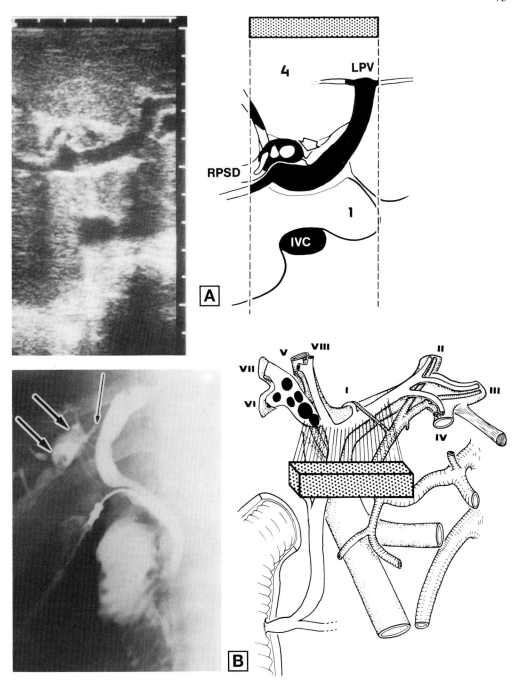

**Fig. 57A, B.** This 20-year-old woman had a cholecystectomy 2 months previously for acute cholecystitis. Operative cholangiogram without high pressure had been considered normal. She was reexplored because of episodes of cholangitis. **A** Operative ultrasound showed an abnormal biliary confluence *(arrow)* with dilatation of a right posterior sectoral duct *(RPSD)*, which was filled with calculi proximal to a stenosis. *LPV*, Left branch of portal vein; *IVC*, inferior vena cava. **B** These findings are seen on a high-pressure cholangiogram, which shows the stenosis *(thin arrow)* with proximal dilatation and calculi *(large arrows)*. *I–VIII* indicate the eight segments of the liver according to Couinaud. Transhepatic horizontal section at the hilus

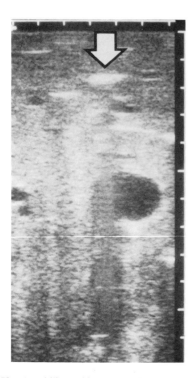

**Fig. 58.** Aerobilia, which can mimic intrahepatic lithiasis, can be distinguished from calculi by its reflected image *(arrow)*, which is larger and narrower with less defined shadowing. This view was obtained after treatment of a stenosis associated with intrahepatic stones. It demonstrates the difficulty of evaluating the completeness of removal of an obstruction by ultrasound because of the artifact produced by aerobilia

## Choledocholithiasis

The role of operative ultrasound in this disease remains the subject of active discussion by clinicians [8, 14, 15].

### Ultrasound Signs of Common Bile Duct Calculi

After the examination of the gallbladder and the intrahepatic bile duct, the extrahepatic bile duct should be examined from the hilus to the papilla. The intrapancreatic portion of the common bile duct is the most difficult to visualize by ultrasound.

Calculi appear as highly echogenic structures with a posterior acoustic shadow the width of which is related to the size of the stone (Fig. 59). Calculi can be generally be identified even in the distal bile duct and the papilla (Fig. 60). A Kocher maneuver, which permits examination posteriorly using the water pouch, can be performed, providing an excellent view of the head of the pancreas and the distal common bile duct.

Dilatation of the common bile duct provides indirect evidence of lithiasis (Fig. 61). The normal duct has a diameter of 4–5 mm, although it can reach 10 mm in elderly patients [11].

The pancreatic parenchyma is normally slightly more echogenic than that of the liver. Foci of pancreatic inflammation which can obstruct the common bile duct or Wirsung's duct can be readily detected by ultrasound (Fig. 62).

Obstruction of the distal common bile duct is often due to neoplastic disease, and this differential diagnosis is crucial to proper therapy. Biliary tumors are generally ill-defined and much less echodense than calculi. They do not have a liquid interface with the duct wall. Diagnostic confirmation requires cholangiography, and in most cases common bile duct exploration is necessary. Operative ultrasound can also improve the accuracy of transduodenal pancreatic needle biopsy, by guiding the biopsy to the most dense area of the lesion.

### Efficacy of Operative Ultrasound in Biliary Disease

The largest series in the literature, from Sigel et al. [13–16] and Jakimowicz et al. [8], include over 200 patients and provide a good reference point in this discussion (Table 2). These results, which compare the sensitivity, specificity, and predictive value of the diagnostic modalities, tend to favor operative ultrasound over cholangiography (Table 3).

The question arises: should operative cholangiography as it is routinely practised

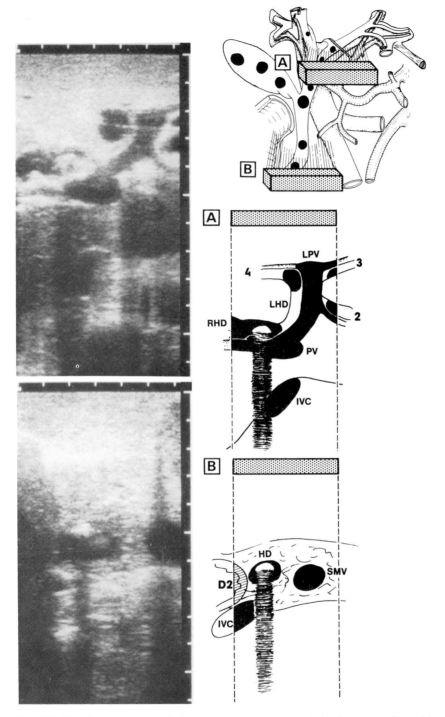

**Fig. 59 A, B.** After an episode of cholangitis, an intravenous cholangiogram performed in this 34-year-old woman revealed multiple stones in the gallbladder and the common bile duct. Operative ultrasound, of which two representative sections, **A** and **B,** are shown, confirmed these findings and showed dilatation of the common bile duct (15 mm). **A** section through the hilus; **B** calculi in the common bile duct. *LPV,* left branch of portal vein, *LHD,* left hepatic duct; *RHD,* right hepatic duct; *PV,* portal vein; *IVC,* inferior vena cava; *HD,* common hepatic duct; *SMV,* superior mesenteric vein; *D2,* second portion of duodenum

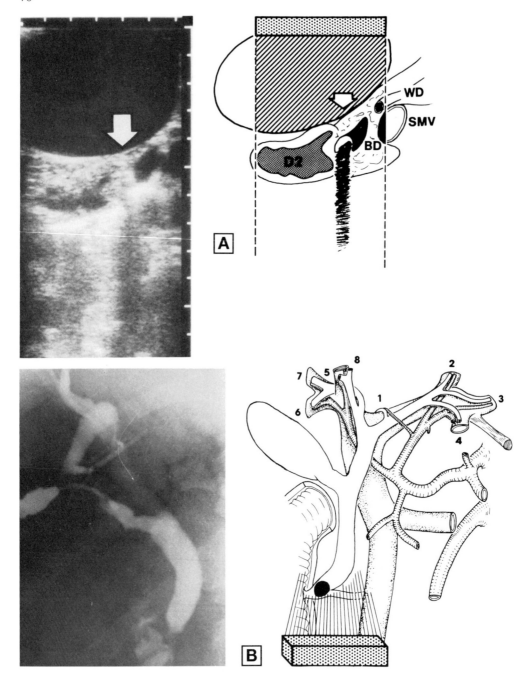

**Fig. 60A, B.** This 48-year-old man presented with a history of several episodes of right upper quadrant pain associated with jaundice and elevated amylase. Preoperatively, ultrasound and intravenous cholangiogram were normal. Intraoperatively, the gallbladder contained no calculi, but had thickened walls and a wide cystic duct. **A** By ultrasound the common bile duct, *(BD)* was of normal caliber (5 mm), with a stone *(arrow)* impacted near the papilla. *SMV,* Superior mesenteric vein; *WD,* Wirsung's duct; *D2,* second portion of duodenum. **B** The stone was seen on fluoroscopy during radiomanometry, but passed with increased pressure, resulting in a normal cholangiogram. Subsequent instrumental examination of the papilla revealed it to be patent. Horizontal section through the head of the pancreas, using the water pouch *(hatched)*

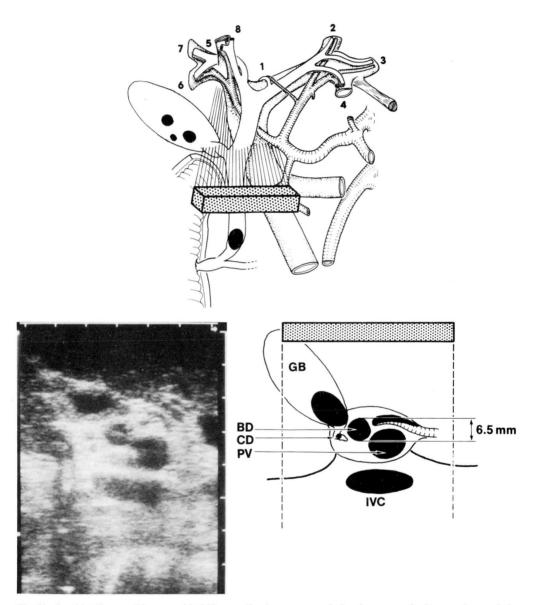

**Fig. 61.** In this 42-year-old man with biliary colic, intravenous cholangiogram and ultrasound revealed cholelithiasis. Operative ultrasound showed the common bile duct to measure 6.5 mm. Cholangiography showed a stone in the distal common bile duct, which was removed on exploration of the duct. *BD*, Common bile duct; *CD*, cystic duct; *PV*, portal vein; *GB*, gallbladder; *IVC*, inferior vena cava. Horizontal section through the hepatoduodenal ligament

be abandoned on the basis of these results? We feel that the key to this issue lies in the quality of the technique of cholangiography which is used in the comparison. Our experience in using a similar technique of cholangiography at the Paul Brousse Hospital between 1970 and 1980 [7] is similar to that reported by Sigel as regards the efficacy of operative ultrasound (Tables 2 and 3). We emphasize that our technique for operative cholangiography includes fluoroscopical examination, manometry, and multiple static views to ensure a complete examination. In contrast, it should be noted that Dr. Sigel's series includes a number of cases in which cholangiography was not performed.

Cholangiography provides precise morphological data and functional information about sphincter of Oddi. Cholangiography is used to confirm the findings of a doubtful ultrasound [8]. Based on these considerations, we fell that good-quality cholangiography remains the best tool for examination of the extrahepatic biliary tree, and that operative ultrasound has as its primary application the detection of intrahepatic lithiasis.

**Table 2.** Results of operative ultrasound compared to cholangiography. Series of Sigel et al. [15], Jakimowicz et al. [8], and the Paul Brousse Hospital (1970–1980) [7]

| | Operative ultrasound | | | | Operative cholangiography | | | | | |
| --- | --- | --- | --- | --- | --- | --- | --- | --- | --- | --- |
| | B. Sigel et al. | | J. Jakimowicz et al. | | B. Sigel et al. | | J. Jakimowicz et al. | | Paul Brousse Hospital | |
| True-positive | 45 | 12.9% | 40 | 20.4% | 30 | 8.6% | 38 | 19.4% | 94 | 18% |
| True-negative | 292 | 83.4% | 147 | 75% | 227 | 64.9% | 134 | 38.4% | 402 | 76.9% |
| False-positive | 4 | 1.1% | 3 | 1.5% | 11 | 3.1% | 10 | 5.1% | 8 | 1.5% |
| False-negative | 3 | 0.9% | 5 | 2.6% | 3 | 0.9% | 6 | 3.1% | 2 | 0.4% |
| Uninterpretable | 5 | 1.4% | 1 | 0.5% | 14 | 4% | 8 | 4.1% | 0 | 0% |
| Not performed | 1 | 0.3% | 0 | 0% | 65 | 18.6% | 0 | 0% | 17 | 3.3% |
| Total | 350 | | 196 | | 350 | | 196 | | 523 | |

**Table 3.** Efficacy (%) of operative ultrasound and cholangiography. Series of Sigel et al. [15], Jakimowicz et al. [8], and the Paul Brousse Hospital (1970–1980) [7]

| | Operative ultrasound | | Cholangiography | | |
| --- | --- | --- | --- | --- | --- |
| | Sigel et al. | Jakimowicz et al. | Sigel et al. | Jakimowicz et al. | Paul Brousse |
| Sensitivity | 93.8 | 89 | 90.9 | 86 | 97.9 |
| Specificity | 98.6 | 98 | 95.4 | 93 | 99 |
| Negative predictive value | 99 | 97 | 98.7 | 96 | 99.5 |
| Positive predictive value | 91 | 93 | 73.2 | 79 | 92 |

## Completion Study After Surgery for Biliary Lithiasis

T-tube cholangiography has generally been used to evaluate the adequacy of a biliary intervention. It is limited in accuracy by several factors, including air bubbles from the procedure, surgical changes, and other artifacts. Unfortunately, ultrasound is no more accurate, since it is also significantly affected by the presence of air bubbles (Fig. 58). Choledochoscopy probably provides the best postoperative study in this situation [5].

## Cholangiocarcinoma

### Ultrasound Signs of Bile Duct Tumors

Examination of these lesions follows the same technique as that in biliary lithiasis. In a systematic fashion the biliary tree is examined, starting with easily identified structures and proceeding toward areas which are more difficult to study. The following information should be obtained in the study:

1. The tumor is first identified as a heterogeneous zone which occupies the lumen of a bile duct and has an echogenicity greater than that of the hepatic parenchyma. The local extent of the tumor is readily identified by ultrasound. In addition, the involvment of the primary and secondary bifurcations of the biliary tree is detected, a fact which has great therapeutic relevance (Fig. 63).
2. Ultrasound readily detects the presence of associated lithiasis.
3. The detection of metastatic spread is facilitated, and can include:

   - Extension into the hepatic parenchyma (for hilar or gallbladder tumors)
   - Invasion of the portal vein (for hilar tumors)
   - Invasion of the hepatoduodenal ligament (for gallbladder tumors)
   - Intrahepatic or nodal metastases

Operative ultrasound also permits the distinction between intrinsic and extrinsic obstruction of the biliary tree (Fig. 64).

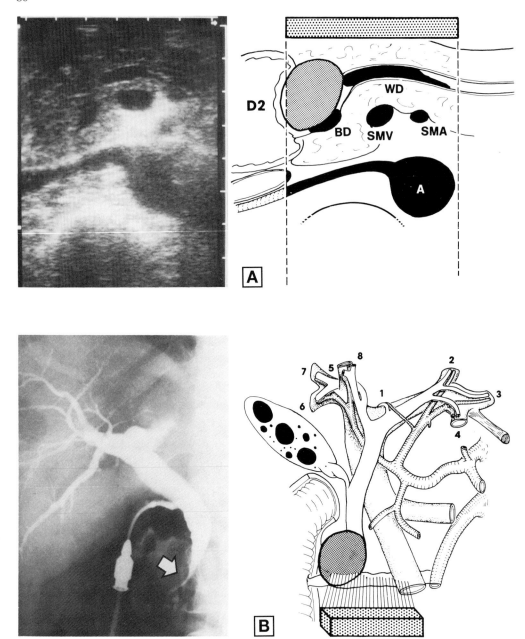

**Fig. 62 A, B.** This 52-year-old man presented with acute pancreatitis and was subsequently found by ultrasound to have microlithiasis of the gallbladder. **A** At operation, ultrasound revealed a focus of pancreatitis in the head near the duct with dilatation of the common bile duct *(BD)* and Wirsung's duct *(WD)*. *SMV,* Superior mesenteric vein; *SMA,* superior mesenteric artery; *A,* aorta and right renal artery. *D2,* second portion of duodenum. **B** Radiomanometry confirmed the presence of a smooth extrinsic compression *(arrow)* of the distal common bile duct. No biopsy was performed and a T-tube was inserted to decompress the biliary tree. A cholangiogram performed 2 months postoperatively was normal, after which the T-tube was removed. One year later the patient remains asymptomatic. Horizontal section through the head of the pancreas

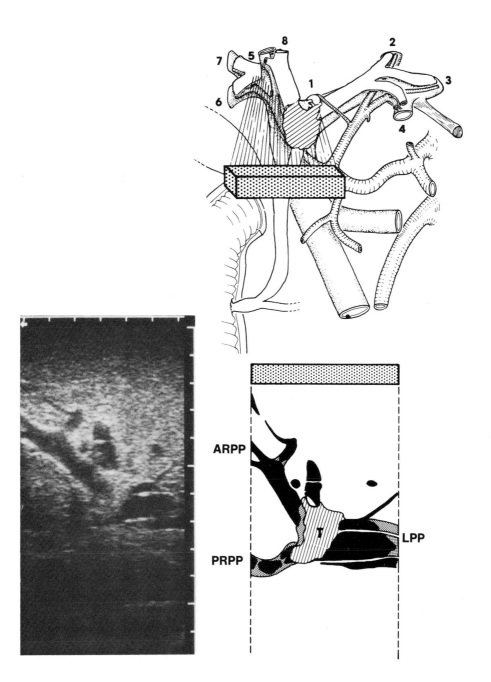

**Fig. 63.** In this 57-year-old man with obstructive jaundice, preoperative ultrasound showed dilatation of the intrahepatic bile ducts and was suggestive of an extrahepatic obtructing lesion. At operation a hilar tumor was found, which was seen by ultrasound to invade the right hepatic duct. The lesion extended to the secondary bifurcation. Right hepatectomy was not possible because of the poor general condition of the patient. Percutaneous cholangiogram was not performed preoperatively, to avoid contamination of the right biliary tree, since it might not be accessible for drainage by a left cholangioenteric anastomosis. *LPP*, left portal pedicle; *ARPP*, anterior right portal pedicle; *PRPP*, posterior right portal pedicle. The area of the tumor *(T)* is indicated by hatching. Horizontal transhepatic section at the hilus

82

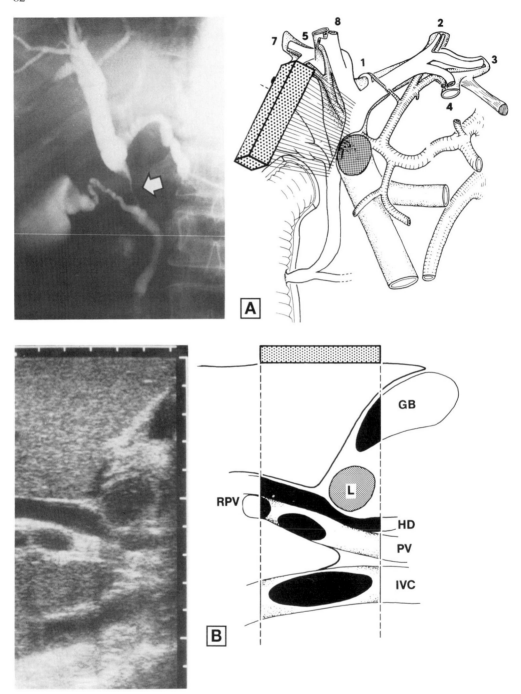

**Fig. 64 A, B.** This 61-year-old man with obstructive jaundice had dilated intrahepatic bile ducts, detected by ultrasound. **A** Percutaneous transhepatic cholangiogram showed a narrowing *(arrow)* of the common hepatic duct *(HD)*. **B** At operation a 2-cm mass involving the hepatic duct was seen and was examined by ultrasound. The lesion was a malignant lymph node of non-Hodgkin's lymphoma, which was removed without opening the bile duct. T-tube drainage was nevertheless established. *L,* lymphadenopathy; *GB,* gallbladder; *PV,* portal vein; *RPV,* right portal vein branch; *IVC,* inferior vena cava. Sagittal transhepatic section along the hepato-duodenal ligament

## Modification of Surgical Tactics

The therapeutic advantage of operative ultrasound rests on several applications:

1. Precise information regarding resectability of the tumor is obtained.
2. Needle biopsy of relevant areas can be readily performed, even for inaccessible lesions.
3. The location of intrahepatic anastomoses can be better planned.
4. Intubation is facilitated.

*Intrahepatic Cholangioenteric Anastomosis.* Formal cholangioenteric anastomosis is usually performed on the bile channel of segment 3, using the round ligament as a landmark for locating the bile duct [2]. In patients with enlarged cholestatic livers, or for access to the right ductal system, operative ultrasound is used to locate a superficial dilated duct. After the duct has been located by ultrasound, it is punctured with a needle and a cholangiogram is performed. If the duct is deemed adequate for the anastomosis, a dye is used to mark the liver to ensure correct placement of the hepatotomy (Fig. 65).

*Ultrasound in Ductal Intubations.* Palliative treatment can be provided by intubation of the proximal ductal system in cases where cholangioenteric anastomosis cannot be performed. The standard approach is to pass the tube blindly through the tumor from below. In contrast, using ultrasound, the duct can be punctured transhepatically, after which a guide wire is passed into position, permitting the precise, atraumatic place of the catheter. This is then left as a internal stent [17], as an external drain, or as a U-tube (for technique see [18]). The efficacy of drainage is increased if a more distal duct is used, and this is more readily accomplished using ultrasound (Fig. 66).

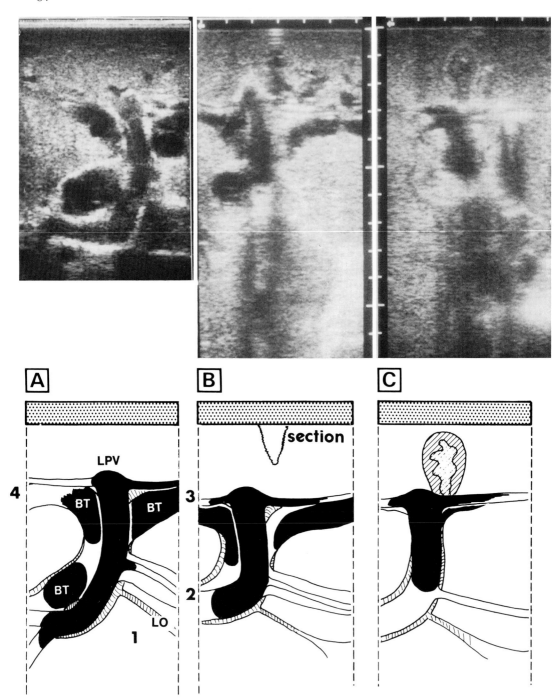

**Fig. 65A–C.** This 56-year-old woman had obstructive jaundice secondary to gallbladder carcinoma invading the hilus of the liver. The tumor was unresectable at operation. **A** Dilatation of the left biliary tree *(BT)*. *LPV*, left portal vein branch; *LO*, lesser omentum. **B** Identification of the bile duct of segment *3*, which is approached through a hepatotomy. **C** Postoperative view of the cholangioenteric anastomosis on the duct of segment *3*. The biliary tree has regained its normal caliber. Horizontal transhepatic sections through the hilus

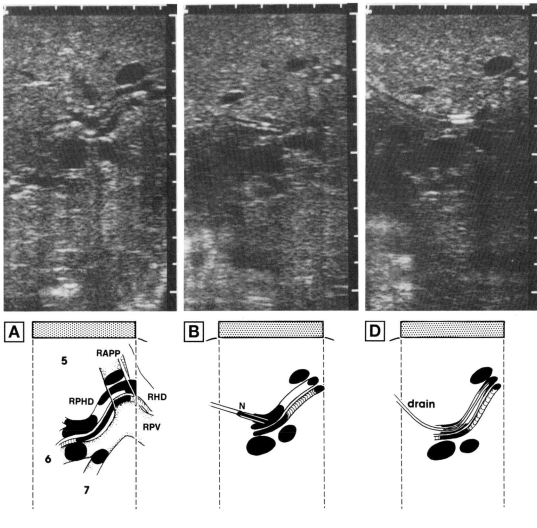

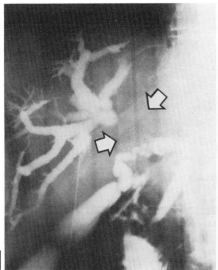

**Fig. 66A–D.** A hilar tumor was found in this 77-year-old woman. At operation the tumor was unresectable. A left intra-hepatic anastomosis was impossible because of the multiple metastatic lesions in the left lobe. **A** On ultrasound the secondary bifurcation seemed to be free. *RPHD*, right posterior hepatic duct; *RAPP*, right anterior portal pedicle; *RPV*, right portal vein branch; *RHD*, right hepatic duct. **B** The biliary tree was punctured (*N*, needle). A cholangiogram performed through the needle (**C**) confirmed these findings and further delineated the anatomy. A small passage of dye through the tumor is seen *(arrows)*. External biliary drainage was established via the needle tract (**D**), since the entire hepatoduodenal ligament was involved with tumor

86

## References

1. Berk RN (1983) Imaging of the gallbladder. In: Moody FG (ed) Advances in diagnosis and surgical treatment of biliary tract disease. Masson, New York, pp 25–39
2. Bismuth H, Corlette MB (1975) Intrahepatic cholangioenteric anastomosis in carcinoma of the hilus of the liver. Surg Gynecol Obstet 140: 170–178
3. Castaing D, Houssin D, Lemoine J, et al (1983) Surgical management of gallstones in cirrhotic patients. Am J Surg 146:310–313
4. Eiseman B, Greenlaw RH, Gallacher JQ (1965) Localization of common duct stones by ultrasound. Arch Surg 91:195–199
5. Grange D, Maillard JN (1981) La cholédochoscopie per-opératoire. Gastroenterol Clin Biol 5:857–865
6. Grüntzig A, Hopff H (1974) Perkutane Rekanalisation chronischer arterieller Verschlüsse mit einem neuen Dilatationskatheter, Modifikation der Dottertechnik. Dtsch Med Wochenschr 99: 2502–2505
7. Hepp J, Bismuth H (1975) Problèmes généraux de la chirurgie de la lithiase biliaire. Techniques chirurgicales. Appareil digestif, Tome 3. Encyclopédie médico-chirurgicale. Paris 40915, 1–16
8. Jakimowicz JJ, Carol EJ, Jürgens PTHJ (1984) The peroperative use of real time B-mode ultrasound imaging in biliary and pancreatic surgery. Dig Surg 1:55–60
9. Knight RP, Newell JA (1963) Operative use of ultrasonics in cholelithiasis. Lancet i:1023–1025
10. Kunstlinger F, Castaing D, Houssin D, et al (1984) Diagnostic échographique des lithiases intra-hépatiques. Gastroenterol Clin Biol 8: 122A
11. Lane RJ, Glazer G (1980) Intra-operative B mode ultrasound scanning of the extra-hepatic biliary system and pancreas. Lancet ii:334–337
12. Niderau C, Sonnenberg A, Mueller J (1984) Comparison of the extra-hepatic bile duct size measured by ultrasound and by different radiographic methods. Gastroenterology 87:615–621
13. Sigel B, Coelho JVC, Spigos DG, et al (1980) Real-time ultrasonography during biliary surgery. Radiology 137:531–533
14. Sigel B (1982) Operative ultrasonography. Lea and Febiger, Philadelphia, pp 53–58
15. Sigel B, Coelho JCV, Nyhus LM, et al (1982) Comparison of cholangiography and ultrasonography in the operative screening of the common bile duct. World J Surg 6:440–444
16. Sigel B, Machii H, Beitler JC, et al (1983) Comparative accuracy of operative ultrasonography and cholangiography in detecting common duct calculi. Surgery 94:715–720
17. Ring EJ, Oleaga JA, Freiman DB, et al (1978) Therapeutic applications of catheter cholangiography. Radiology, 128:333–338
18. Praderi R, Mazza M, Gomez Possatj C, Estefan A (1974) Le drainage transhépatique en séton. Nouv Presse Medicale 3:2015–2018

# 4 Operative Ultrasound
# in the Surgery of Portal Hypertension

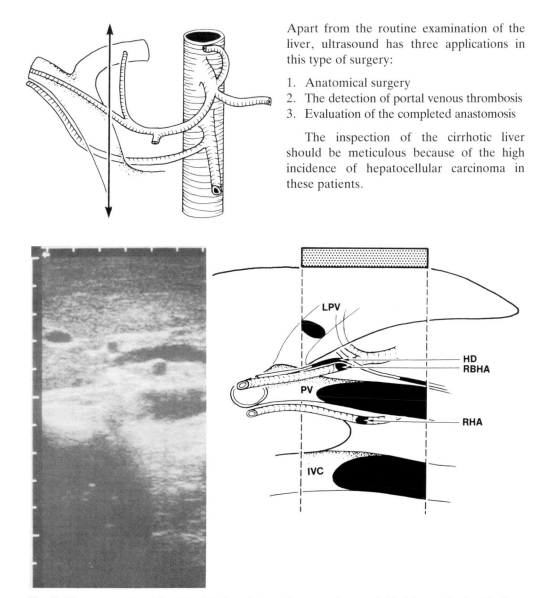

Apart from the routine examination of the liver, ultrasound has three applications in this type of surgery:

1. Anatomical surgery
2. The detection of portal venous thrombosis
3. Evaluation of the completed anastomosis

The inspection of the cirrhotic liver should be meticulous because of the high incidence of hepatocellular carcinoma in these patients.

**Fig. 67.** When a separate origin of the right hepatic artery is present, it passes behind the portal vein at the base of the hepatoduodenal ligament to enter the right border of the hilus. The presence of this arterial anomaly interferes with the mobilization of the portal vein, which is essential to the creation of a side-to-side portacaval shunt. *LPV*, left branch of portal vein; *HD*, common hepatic duct; *RBHA*, right branch of hepatic artery; *PV*, portal vein; *RHA*, right hepatic artery; *IVC*, inferior vena cava. Sagittal transhepatic section, centred on hepatic ligament

88

## Anatomical Exploration

The portal vein can quite easily be localized without ultrasound. The identification of aberrant arterial anatomy which could interfere with the realization of side-to-side portacaval anastomosis is the most important application of ultrasound [1] (Fig. 67).

Operative ultrasound is probably more useful in other types of shunt, for example:

Localization of the renal vein in splenorenal anastomosis [2].

When using an extraperitoneal approach for splenorenal anastomosis, the dissection can be reduced by using ultrasound for localization of the vessels [3].

Since the superior mesenteric vein is often surrounded by fat and lymph nodes [4], its localization for mesocaval shunting can be facilitated by operative ultrasound (Fig. 68).

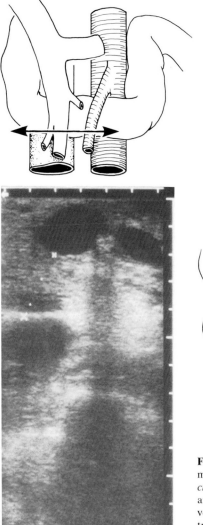

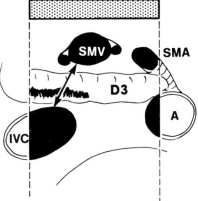

**Fig. 68.** Localization of the superior mesenteric vein *(SMV)* for a mesocaval shunt. The distance between the *two arrows* (*two crosses* on ultrasound image) is 2.5 cm. *SMA,* superior mesenteric artery; *D3,* third portion of the duodenum; *A,* aorta; *IVC,* inferior vena cava. Horizontal section with the probe on the root of the transverse mesocolon

## Detection of Portal Vein Thrombosis

Operative ultrasound is often better than arteriography in the detection of partial portal thrombosis. The walls of the portal vein are clearly seen by ultrasound.

## Evaluation of Completed Anastomoses

Operative ultrasound permits measurement of the size of the anastomosis. An assessment of flow is obtained by the detection of moving echoes in the lumen (Fig. 69).

## References

1. Bismuth H (1906) Les anastomoses porto-caves tronculaires. Encycl Med Chir, Paris, Techniques chirurgicales. Appareil digestif 40805
2. Bismuth H, Moreaux J, Hepp J (1966) L'anastomose splénorénale centrale dans le traitement de l'hypertension portale. Ann Chir 20:1441–1445
3. Stoney RJ, Mehigan JT, Olcott C (1975) Retroperitoneal approach for portasystemic decompression. Arch Surg 110:1347–1350
4. Drapanas T (1972) Interposition mesocaval shunt for treatment of portal hypertension. Ann Surg 176:435–447

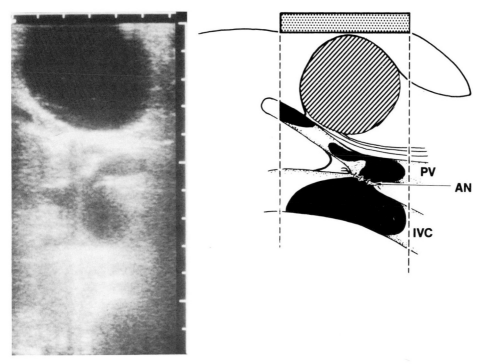

**Fig. 69.** This 65-year-old man with postnecrotic cirrhosis presented with a history of multiple episodes of gastrointestinal bleeding from esophageal varices. A side-to-side portacaval anastomosis was performed, which is visualized by ultrasound using the water pouch *(hatched)*. Flow across the anastomosis *(AN)* is clearly visible. *PV,* portal vein; *IVC,* inferior vena cava

# Conclusion

Reviewing the results of 2 years of intense, daily application of operative ultrasound in the practice of hepatobiliary surgery, we are able to make some comments about its utility.

In hepatic surgery, ultrasound clearly fulfils its potential. Using this technique, the surgeon can localize the lesion within the liver, identify metastatic extension, and precisely define vascular anatomy. The surgeon, who was previously dependent upon external landmarks and palpation, can now proceed more confidently in the surgical treatment of liver disease. The organ becomes "transparent" with ultrasound, a development which must be considered truly revolutionary.

In biliary surgery, ultrasound competes with operative cholangiography, which is a technique of proven efficacy. Ultrasound is clearly of benefit in the detection of intrahepatic lithiasis; however, its utility in the surgery of extrahepatic lithiasis is probably dependent on the quality of cholangiography practised by the biliary surgeon.

Several questions about the role of operative ultrasound in digestive surgery remain to be answered:
The role of ultrasound in pancreatic disease
Its utility in the treatment of portal hypertension
The consequences of the detection of small hepatic metastases in gastrointestinal tract tumors both in terms of immediate operative management and eventual prognosis. This issue may eventually result in the routine use of ultrasound for scanning the liver during laparotomy for gastrointestinal malignancy.

The present work must be considered as only an introduction to the use of operative ultrasound in digestive surgery. With continued improvements in ultrasound technology and widening clinical experience, the true benefit of operative ultrasound will be appreciated.